Suicide in Children and Adolescents

This book highlights the current epidemiology of suicide among children and adolescents, as well as identifying important risk factors and evidence-based treatment options. To accomplish this, this book is organized into two major sections: (1) contributing factors to the emergence of child and adolescent suicide, and (2) evidence-based treatment of child and adolescent suicide.

Across studies, researchers discuss risk factors of anxiety, sleep problems, child sexual abuse, and violence perpetration, and conclude with treatment considerations including the Collaborative Assessment and Management of Suicidality (CAMS) and safety planning. From this body of work, it is clear that there is an urgent need to better understand and effectively treat child and adolescent suicide. The book will be a great resource for academics, researchers, and advanced students of Psychology, Psychiatry, Medicine, Sociology, Social Work, and Youth Studies.

The chapters in this book were originally published as a special issue of *Children's Health Care*.

Michelle A. Patriquin, PhD, ABPP, is Director of Research at The Menninger Clinic and is Associate Professor in the Department of Psychiatry and Behavioral Sciences at Baylor College of Medicine. She is board certified by the American Board of Professional Psychology (ABPP) in clinical child and adolescent psychology.

Katrina A. Rufino, PhD, is Associate Professor of Psychology at the University of Houston-Downtown in the Department of Social Sciences. She is also a senior data scientist and the principal investigator for suicide-related projects at the Menninger Clinic.

Suicide in Children and Adolescents

New Interventions and Risk Factors

Edited by
Michelle A. Patriquin and Katrina A. Rufino

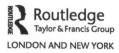

LONDON AND NEW YORK

First published 2022
by Routledge
2 Park Square, Milton Park, Abingdon, Oxon OX14 4RN

and by Routledge
605 Third Avenue, New York, NY 10158

Routledge is an imprint of the Taylor & Francis Group, an informa business

© 2022 Taylor & Francis

British Library Cataloguing in Publication Data
A catalogue record for this book is available from the British Library

ISBN: 978-1-032-05840-5 (hbk)
ISBN: 978-1-032-05841-2 (pbk)
ISBN: 978-1-003-19945-8 (ebk)

Typeset in Minion Pro
by Newgen Publishing UK

Publisher's Note
The publisher accepts responsibility for any inconsistencies that may have arisen during the conversion of this book from journal articles to book chapters, namely the inclusion of journal terminology.

Disclaimer
Every effort has been made to contact copyright holders for their permission to reprint material in this book. The publishers would be grateful to hear from any copyright holder who is not here acknowledged and will undertake to rectify any errors or omissions in future editions of this book.

Contents

Citation Information

The chapters in this book were originally published in the *Children's Health Care*, volume 48, issue 4 (2019). When citing this material, please use the original page numbering for each article, as follows:

Chapter 1

Child and adolescent suicide: contributing risk factors and new evidence-based interventions
Katrina A. Rufino and Michelle A. Patriquin
Children's Health Care, volume 48, issue 4 (2019), pp. 345–350

Chapter 2

The role of anxiety for youth experiencing suicide-related behaviors
Darby Covert and Maria G. Fraire
Children's Health Care, volume 48, issue 4 (2019), pp. 351–371

Chapter 3

Sleep patterns and anxiety in children interact to predict later suicidal ideation
Priel Meir, Candice A. Alfano, Simon Lau, Ryan M. Hill, and Cara A. Palmer
Children's Health Care, volume 48, issue 4 (2019), pp. 372–393

Chapter 4

An examination of the interactive effects of different types of childhood abuse and perceived social support on suicidal ideation
Laura C. Wilson, Amie R. Newins, and Nathan A. Kimbrel
Children's Health Care, volume 48, issue 4 (2019), pp. 394–409

Chapter 5

Violent victimization and perpetration as distinct risk factors for adolescent suicide attempts
Evan E. Rooney, Ryan M. Hill, Benjamin Oosterhoff, and Julie B. Kaplow
Children's Health Care, volume 48, issue 4 (2019), pp. 410–427

Chapter 6

Establishing a research agenda for child and adolescent safety planning
Christopher W. Drapeau
Children's Health Care, volume 48, issue 4 (2019), pp. 428–443

Chapter 7

The potential use of CAMS for suicidal youth: building on epidemiology and clinical interventions
David A. Jobes, Genesis A. Vergara, Elizabeth C. Lanzillo, and Abby Ridge-Anderson
Children's Health Care, volume 48, issue 4 (2019), pp. 444–468

For any permission-related enquiries please visit:
www.tandfonline.com/page/help/permissions

Notes on Contributors

Candice A. Alfano, Department of Psychology, University of Houston, Houston, TX, USA.

Darby Covert, Franciscan Children's, Brighton, MA, USA.

Christopher W. Drapeau, Department of Health Policy and Management, Richard M. Fairbanks School of Public Health, Indiana University, Indianapolis, IN, USA; Division of Mental Health and Addiction, Indiana Family and Social Services Administration, Indianapolis, IN, USA.

Maria G. Fraire, Franciscan Children's, Brighton, MA, USA; McLean Hospital, Harvard Medical School, Brighton, MA, USA.

Ryan M. Hill, Department of Pediatrics, Baylor College of Medicine/Texas Children's Hospital, Houston, TX, USA.

David A. Jobes, Department of Psychology, The Catholic University of America, Washington, DC, USA.

Julie B. Kaplow, Hackett Center for Mental Health, Houston, TX, USA.

Nathan A. Kimbrel, Department of Psychiatry and Behavioral Sciences, Duke University Medical Center, Durham, NC, USA; Durham VA Medical Center, Durham, NC, USA; VA Mid- Atlantic Mental Illness Research, Education, and Clinical Center, Durham, NC, USA.

Elizabeth C. Lanzillo, Department of Psychology, The Catholic University of America, Washington, DC, USA.

Simon Lau, Department of Psychology, University of Houston, Houston, TX, USA.

Priel Meir, Department of Psychology, University of Houston, Houston, TX, USA.

Amie R. Newins, Department of Psychology, University of Central Florida, Orlando, FL, USA.

Benjamin Oosterhoff, Department of Psychology, Montana State University, Bozeman, MT, USA.

Cara A. Palmer, Department of Psychology, Montana State University, Bozeman, MT, USA.

Michelle A. Patriquin, The Menninger Clinic, Houston, TX, USA; Menninger Department of Psychiatry and Behavioral Sciences, Baylor College of Medicine, Houston, TX, USA; Michael E. DeBakey VA Medical Center, Houston, TX, USA.

Abby Ridge-Anderson, Department of Psychology, The Catholic University of America, Washington, DC, USA.

Evan E. Rooney, Department of Pediatrics, Baylor College of Medicine/Texas Children's Hospital, Houston, TX, USA.

Katrina A. Rufino, The Menninger Clinic, Houston, TX, USA; Menninger Department of Psychiatry and Behavioral Sciences, Baylor College of Medicine, Houston, TX, USA; Department of Social Sciences, The University of Houston Downtown, Houston, TX, USA.

Genesis A. Vergara, Department of Psychology, The Catholic University of America, Washington, DC, USA.

Laura C. Wilson, Department of Psychological Science, University of Mary Washington, Fredericksburg, VA, USA.

Child and adolescent suicide: contributing risk factors and new evidence-based interventions

Katrina A. Rufino and Michelle A. Patriquin

ABSTRACT

Our goal of this special issue is to detail and describe the current epidemiology of suicide among children and adolescents, as well as highlight important risk factors and evidence-based treatment options. To accomplish this, our issue is organized in two major sections: (1) contributing factors to the emergence of child and adolescent suicide, and (2) evidence-based treatment of child and adolescent suicide. Within the issue, authors discuss risk factors of anxiety, sleep problems, child sexual abuse, and violence perpetration, and conclude with treatment considerations including the Collaborative Assessment and Management of Suicidality (CAMS) and safety planning. Across studies, it is clear that there is an urgent need to better understand and effectively treat child and adolescent suicide.

Introduction

Current Centers for Disease Control and Prevention (CDC) data indicate that suicide is the second leading cause of death for both children and adolescents ages 10 to 17, second to only unintentional injury (CDC, 2017). This statistic is evidence of rising rates of suicide among children and adolescents, as ten years prior, suicide was the fourth leading cause of death among children ages 10 to 17 (CDC, 2017). Furthermore, suicide is now the 9th leading cause of death among children ages 5 to 11 (CDC, 2017). Unfortunately, these death statistics comport with recent literature which found a 92% increase in annual emergency department (ED) visits for suicide ideation and attempts from 2007 to 2015 for children under the age of 18, despite no statistically significant increase in the overall number of ED visits (Burstein, Agostino, & Greenfield, 2019). Those admitted to the ED for a suicide attempt increased by 79% from 2007 to 2015, and almost half (43.1%) of all ED visits for suicide ideation or a suicide attempt were for children between the ages of 5 and 10 (Burstein et al., 2019).

The rising rates of suicide attempts and death, particularly in younger children, indicate the urgent need to develop a better understanding of contributing risk factors to increased suicide risk and to design new evidence-based interventions for suicide in children and adolescents. As such, our special issue is organized in two sections: (1) papers that highlight contributing risk factors of increased suicide risk and (2) papers describing new treatments for suicide in children and adolescents.

Contributing risk factors to child & adolescent suicide

In order to effectively prevent and intervene, it is critical to build an empirically-based conceptualization of the contributing factors that increase child and adolescent suicide. In this section on contributing risk factors, the authors review unique factors that increase suicide risk including anxiety, sleep problems, child sexual abuse, and violent victimization. Notably, there are other factors that are not included in the present issue that also contribute to increased risk (e.g., seasonal trends with higher rates of suicide attempts in the school year, self-harm; Carbone, Holzer, & Vaughn, 2019).

To begin the special issue and open the section on risk factors, Covert and Fraire (2019) provide a comprehensive review of the literature on how specific anxiety disorders may serve as risk factors for suicide-related behavior in youth. An important take away from their review, is the relative lack of research on the role of anxiety disorders and suicide in youth. They conclude that social anxiety disorder appears to have the most developed literature, with the presence of social anxiety disorder related to increased risk for suicide-related behavior in adolescents. Additionally, generalized anxiety disorder also serves as a risk factor for suicidal behavior in adolescents. Importantly, the Covert and Fraire (2019) article makes a relevant clinical suggestion: when determining a child or adolescent's suicide risk, we should not only be examining this within the context of depression – which is most commonly done in clinical practice – but also anxiety disorders, particularly given their high comorbidity with depression.

Given the importance of understanding the role of anxiety in suicide, a natural extension of this work is to examine how sleep problems relate to anxiety and suicide. Sleep problems are one of the most powerful, but understudied, predictors of all suicide outcomes – ideation, attempt, and death (Glenn et al., 2018). Moreover, sleep problems are highly prevalent in youth with anxiety disorders (Alfano, Patriquin, & De Los Reyes, 2015; Cowie et al., 2014; Patriquin, Mellman, Glaze, & Alfano, 2014). In the second paper in this special issue, Meir and colleagues (2019) present empirical findings from a longitudinal study on sleep and anxiety that demonstrate that children with greater anxiety are at higher risk of future suicidal ideation when there are childhood sleep disturbances and high percentages of rapid eye movement (REM) sleep present in early childhood. Their study indicates that the assessment of anxiety is important in clinical practice for determining suicide risk, but so is the assessment of sleep problems.

Outside these emerging new risk factors for suicide in youth, trauma is a well-studied risk factor particularly physical, emotional, and sexual abuse, and physical neglect (Zatti et al., 2017). The third paper in this section by Wilson and colleagues (2019) provides new evidence that examines the interaction between the types of childhood abuse and social support in relation to adulthood suicide ideation in female survivors of childhood sexual abuse or physical abuse. Their findings suggest that family and friend support may be especially helpful in supporting women who have experienced childhood sexual abuse to in turn reduce their risk of developing suicidal ideation in adulthood.

The last paper in this section by Rooney and colleagues (2019) extends the examination of traumatic events and suicide, by assessing the association between violent victimization and perpetration and suicide attempts. Using a sample of youth who previously experienced suicidal ideation, they examined the role of acquired capability via violent victimization and perpetration (Van Orden et al., 2010). Rooney and colleagues (2019) discuss new developmental conceptualizations of suicide risk and interesting clinical implications for practitioners working with adolescents including the regular assessment of trauma history and both violent and nonviolent externalizing behaviors.

Evidence-based treatment of child & adolescent suicide

In light of the increased rates of suicide among children and adolescents, the importance of suicide treatment for youth is apparent now more than ever. Recent studies have determined the efficacy of treatments adapted for youth from the adult literature for reducing suicide risk: Dialectical Behavior Therapy (DBT; McCauley et al., 2018; Mehlum et al., 2016, 2014), Cognitive Behavioral Therapy for Suicide Prevention (CBT-SP; Alavi, Sharifi, Ghanizadeh, & Dehbozorgi, 2013), Mentalization Based Therapy for Adolescents (MBT-A; Roussouw & Fonagy, 2012), and combinations thereof, such as Safe Alternatives for Teens and Youths (SAFETY; Asarnow, Hughes, Babeva, & Sugar, 2017) which is informed by both CBT and DBT. DBT studies demonstrate that while initial gains are strong leading to significant differences between groups (McCauley et al., 2018; Mehlum et al., 2014), follow-up at one year shows that the initial advantage of DBT for youth diminishes (McCauley et al., 2018; Mehlum et al., 2016) showing the strength of DBT for youth in a suicidal crisis, but also a need for the continued reinforcement of DBT skills. While both CBT-SP (Alavi et al., 2013) and MBT-A (Roussouw & Fonagy, 2012) have demonstrated significant improvement in suicide risk over the course of treatment compared to treatment as usual, neither study included follow-up after the conclusion of treatment to determine if treatment gains were sustained. Our special issue adds to this literature by reviewing two new treatments for youth, CAMS and safety planning.

First, Jobes and colleagues (2019) provide an in depth look at existing evidence-based interventions for the treatment of suicidal children and adolescents. They provide a thorough review of the epidemiology of prevalence rates and possible risk factors including childhood trauma, bullying, academic pressure, psychopathology, and biological factors. Additionally, Jobes and colleagues (2019) discuss the adaptation of CAMS, an already established evidenced-based suicide intervention for adults (Andreasson et al., 2016; Comtois et al., 2011; Ellis, Rufino, Allen, Fowler, & Jobes, 2015; Huh et al., 2018), for children and teens, as well as current studies showing support for its use with these populations. Jobes and colleagues (2019) indicate the preliminary evidence for the psychometrics of the SSF with youth and discuss the ongoing effectiveness studies currently in place for a youth version of CAMS.

The last paper of this special issue by Drapeau (2019) discusses the use of safety planning with suicidal patients as well as the research support for the practice in both adults and youth. He then examines the need for further research specific to safety planning with children and adolescents, and the unique hurdles that may be presented with this population, specifically the parent-professional collaboration. Novel applications of safety planning with youth are discussed and the author concludes with suggestions for clinicians, like adaptation for cognitive ability or involving parents.

Conclusion

The rates of suicide deaths and attempts in children and adolescents continue to rise. In this special issue, the contributing papers find that the significant pain experienced by these children and adolescents is related to multiple risk factors including anxiety, sleep problems, and trauma. It is our hope that understanding new risk factors for suicide in youth will lead to the design of novel interventions and treatments, such as the youth version of CAMS and new safety planning methods. Through innovative evidence-based solutions to youth suicide, clinical science and mental health care professionals can provide these children and their families some relief from their pain and, eventually, reverse the climbing rates of suicide in children and adolescents.

Disclosure statement

No potential conflict of interest was reported by the authors.

Funding

This work was supported by the The Menninger Clinic Foundation.

References

Alavi, A., Sharifi, B., Ghanizadeh, A., & Dehbozorgi, G. (2013). Effectiveness of cognitive-behavioral therapy in decreasing suicidal ideation and hopelessness of the adolescents with previous suicidal attempts. *Iran Journal of Pediatrics, 23*, 467–472.

Alfano, C. A., Patriquin, M. A., & De Los Reyes, A. (2015). Subjective–Objective sleep comparisons and discrepancies among clinically-anxious and healthy children. *Journal of Abnormal Child Psychology, 43*(7), 1343–1353. doi:10.1007/s10802-015-0018-7

Andreasson, K., Krogh, J., Wenneberg, C., Jessen, H. K. L., Krakauer, K., Gluud, C., & Nordentoft, M. (2016). Effectiveness of dialectical behavior therapy versus collaborative assessment and management of suicidality treatment for reduction of self-harm in adults with borderline personality disorder – A randomized observer-blinded clinical trial. *Depression and Anxiety, 33*, 520–530. doi:10.1002/da.22472

Asarnow, J. R., Hughes, J. L., Babeva, K. N., & Sugar, C. A. (2017). Cognitive-behavioral family treatment for suicide attempt prevention: A randomized controlled trial. *Journal of the American Academy of Child and Adolescent Psychiatry, 56*, 506–514. doi:10.1016/j.jaac.2017.03.015

Burstein, B., Agostino, H., & Greenfield, B. (2019). Suicidal attempts and ideation among children and adolescents in US emergency departments, 2007-2015. *JAMA Pediatrics, 173*, 598. doi:10.1001/jamapediatrics.2019.0464

Carbone, J. T., Holzer, K. J., & Vaughn, M. G. (2019). Child and adolescent suicidal ideation and suicide attempts: Evidence from the healthcare cost and utilization project. *The Journal of Pediatrics, 206*, 225–231. doi:10.1016/j.jpeds.2018.10.017

Centers for Disease Control and Prevention (CDC). (2017). *Web-based Injury statistics query and reporting system.* Retrieved from https://www.cdc.gov/injury/wisqars/fatal.html

Comtois, K. A., Jobes, D. A., O'Connor, S., Atkins, D. C., Janis, K., Chessen, C., … Youdelis Flores, C. (2011). Collaborative assessment and management of suicidality (CAMS): Feasibility trial for next-day appointment services. *Depression and Anxiety, 28*, 963–972. doi:10.1002/da.20895

Covert, D., & Fraire, M. G. (2019). The role of anxiety for youth experiencing suicide-related behaviors. *Children's Health Care, 48*(4), 351–371.

Cowie, J., Alfano, C. A., Patriquin, M. A., Reynolds, K. C., Talavera, D., & Clementi, M. A. (2014). Addressing sleep in children with anxiety disorders. *Sleep Medicine Clinics, 9*(2), 137–148. doi:10.1016/j.jsmc.2014.02.001

Drapeau, C. W. (2019). Establishing a research agenda for child and adolescent safety planning. *Children's Health Care, 48*(4), 428–443.

Ellis, T. E., Rufino, K. A., Allen, J. G., Fowler, J. C., & Jobes, D. A. (2015). Impact of a suicide-specific intervention within inpatient psychiatric care: The collaborative assessment and management of suicidality. *Suicide and Life Threatening Behavior, 45*, 556–566. doi:10.1111/sltb.12151

Glenn, C. R., Kleiman, E. M., Cha, C. B., Deming, C. A., Franklin, J. C., & Nock, M. K. (2018). Understanding suicide risk within the Research Domain Criteria (RDoC) framework: A meta-analytic review. *Depression and Anxiety, 35*(1), 65–88. doi:10.1002/da.22686

Huh, D., Jobes, D. A., Comtois, K. A., Kerbrat, A. H., Chalker, S. A., Gutierrez, P. M., & Jennings, K. W. (2018). The Collaborative Assessment and Management of Suicidality

(CAMS) versus Enhanced Care as Usual (E-CAU) with suicidal soldiers: Moderator analyses from a randomized controlled trial. *Military Psychology, 30,* 495–506. doi:10.1080/08995605.2018.1503001

Jobes, D. A., Vergara, G. A., Lanzillo, E. C., & Ridge-Andersen, A. (2019). Clinical suicide prevention for adolescents and children: The epidemiology of the problem, clinical interventions to date, and the potential use of CAMS for suicidal youth. *Children's Health Care, 48*(4), 444–468.

McCauley, E., Berk, M. S., Asarnow, J. R., Adrian, M., Cohen, J., Korslund, K., ... Linehan, M. M. (2018). Efficacy of dialectical behavior therapy for adolescents at high risk for suicide: A randomized clinical trial. *JAMA Psychiatry, 75,* 777–785. doi:10.1001/jamapsychiatry.2018.1109

Mehlum, L., Ramberg, M., Tormoen, A. J., Haga, E., Diep, L. M., Stanley, B. H., ... Grøholt, B. (2016). Dialectical behavior therapy compared with enhanced usual care over adolescents with repeated suicidal and self-harming behavior: Outcomes over a one-year follow-up. *Journal of the Academy of Child and Adolescent Psychiatry, 55,* 295–300. doi:10.1016/j.jaac.2016.01.005

Mehlum, L., Tormoen, A. J., Ramberg, M., Haga, E., Diep, L. M., Laberg, S., ... Grøholt, B. (2014). Dialectic behavior therapy for adolescents with repeated suicidal and self-harming behavior: A randomized trial. *Journal of the American Academy of Child and Adolescent Psychiatry, 53,* 1082–1091. doi:10.1016/j.jaac.2014.07.003

Meir, P., Alfano, C. A., Lau, S., Hill, R. M., & Palmer, C. A. (2019). Sleep patterns and anxiety in children interact to predict later suicidal ideation. *Children's Health Care, 48*(4), 372–393.

Patriquin, M. A., Mellman, T. A., Glaze, D. G., & Alfano, C. A. (2014). Polysomnographic sleep characteristics of generally-anxious and healthy children assessed in the home environment. *Journal of Affective Disorders, 161*(1), 79–83. doi:10.1016/j.jad.2014.02.037

Rooney, E. E., Hill, R. M., Oosterhoff, B., & Kaplow, J. B. (2019). Violent victimization and perpetration as distinct risk factors for adolescent suicide attempts. *Children's Health Care, 48*(4), 410–427. doi:10.1080/02739615.2019.1630280

Roussouw, T. I., & Fonagy, P. (2012). Mentalization-based treatment for self-harm in adolescents: A randomized controlled trial. *Journal of the American Academy of Child and Adolescent Psychiatry, 51,* 1304–1313. doi:10.1016/j.jaac.2012.09.018

Van Orden, K. A., Witte, T. K., Cukrowicz, K. C., Braithwaite, S. R., Selby, E. A., & Joiner, T. E. (2010). The interpersonal theory of suicide. *Psychological Review, 117,* 575–600. doi:10.1037/a0018697

Wilson, L. C., Newins, A. R., & Kimbrel, N. A. (2019). An examination of the interactive effects of different types of childhood abuse and perceived social support on suicidal ideation. *Children's Health Care, 48*(4), 394–409.

Zatti, C., Rosa, V., Barros, A., Valdivia, L., Calegaro, V. C., Freitas, L. H., ... Schuch, F. B. (2017). Childhood trauma and suicide attempt: A meta-analysis of longitudinal studies from the last decade. *Psychiatry Research, 256,* 353–358. doi:10.1016/j.psychres.2017.06.082

The role of anxiety for youth experiencing suicide-related behaviors

Darby Covert and Maria G. Fraire

ABSTRACT

The primary aim of this review is to explore how anxiety, and specific anxiety disorders, may be risk factors for suicide-related behavior in youth. Findings from adult literature are presented to serve as a foundation but highlighted as inadequate to replace the needed research specifically tailored to youth. Preliminary evidence for anxiety as a risk factor to suicidal behaviors in youth exists but is not well studied or understood. Suggestions for future research and clinical implications of relevant findings are presented for consideration.

Currently, suicide is the second leading cause of death amongst individuals ages 10–34; claiming the lives of over 400 children ages 10–14 annually (Centers for Disease Control, 2018). The aim of this review is to explore the relationship of anxiety disorders as a risk factor for suicide-related behaviors in children and adolescents. Specifically, examining anxiety as a construct in children as well as expand upon the current literature in order to speak to more specific diagnoses. The comorbidity between anxiety and depression is discussed as it does play a role in the complexity of anxiety as a risk factor. Through the analysis of existing literature, the lack of emphasis on the population of youth is apparent and calls for further exploration. To this end, a brief review of adult orientated literature is also included, as more research has been conducted looking at specific anxiety disorders and suicide risks in adults. The implications for future practice focusing on anxiety in relation to suicide-related behaviors have great potential.

Suicide-related behaviors are classified as suicidal ideation, non-fatal suicide attempts, and suicide (Silverman, Berman, Sanddal, O'Carroll, & Joiner, 2007). Suicidal ideation refers to an individual's self-reported thoughts, consideration or planning of killing oneself. A suicide attempt is a non-fatal, self-directed, potentially injurious act with the intent to die as a result of said act. Suicide refers to self-inflicted injurious behavior with implicit intent to die and does subsequently end in death (National Institute of Mental Health, 2018). On average, there are 123 completed suicides daily in the United

States alone, surmounting to nearly 50,000 deaths annually (American Foundation for Suicide Prevention, 2015). In 2016, suicide was the 10th leading cause of death amongst individuals in the United States, a rate that has steadily increased over recent years. The suicide rate increased 30% from 2000–2016, increasing on average by 1% annually from the years 2000 to 2006 and increasing by 2% annually from 2006 through 2016 (Centers for Disease Control, 2018).

Specifically, suicide rates were found to be significantly higher amongst individuals ages 10–24 in 2016 compared to rates from this population in 2000. While this population may not be regarded as frequently engaging in suicide-related behaviors, data indicates these behaviors are prevalent. Reported in the Youth Risk Behaviors Study (2018), 8.6% of adolescents in high school (grades 9–12) reported at least one suicide attempt in the last 12 months. Research suggests self-reports of younger children (ages 7–12) who attempt suicide share similarities with older children and adolescents regarding suicide-related behavior. Relationships were not affected by age, gender or race (Bodzy, Barreto, Swenson, Liguori, & Costea, 2016). This suggests that applicable differences regarding suicide-related behavior between these given categories identified in adults may not be developed in youth. Unfortunately, the literature focusing on this younger population regarding suicide-related behavior is still in the early stages compared to the adult literature. Given some findings are able to compare differences between adult and youth suicidal behaviors, existing research found amongst older populations could inform, but not completely explain, behaviors in children and adolescents. Enhancing our understanding of children who are engaging in suicide-related behavior is incredibly important, given that children are likely to continue engaging in similar behaviors into their adolescent and adult years. While younger groups (i.e. ages 15–24) have consistently had lower suicide rates when compared to middle-aged or older adults (American Foundation for Suicide Prevention, 2018), literature support risk factors developing within this adolescent age range (Olatunji, Cisler, & Tolin, 2007).

Risk factors for suicide-related behavior

Given the paucity of research in suicidal behaviors in youth, compared to the body of research in suicidal behaviors in adults, a review of the adult literature serves as a springboard to begin to understand suicidal behaviors as a whole. Substantial research has been conducted in order to identify risk factors associated with suicide-related behavior in adults. Research suggests that the most significant risk factor for suicide is a previous suicide attempt (Malone, Haas, Sweeney, & Mann, 1995). Well-studied examples of risk factors include impulsivity, a tendency for pessimism, hopelessness, perceiving fewer reasons for living, and chronic substance abuse (Brodsky et al.,

2001). Additionally, a family history of psychiatric disorders, a previous suicide attempt, severe depression, hopelessness, comorbid disorders (including anxiety), and substance abuse were all found to be risk factors for suicide amongst an adult population (Hawton, Comabella, Haw, & Saunders, 2013).

Developing a better understanding of suicidal behaviors in adolescents is a burgeoning research area. Psychological autopsies of adolescent suicide victims yielded results indicating a high prevalence of mental disorders among young suicide victims (Portzky, Audenaert, & van Heeringen, 2009). A family history of suicide, a family history of child maltreatment, a previous suicide attempt, a history of mental illness (specifically depression), a history of alcohol and substance abuse, feelings of hopelessness, impulsive or aggressive behavior, local epidemics of suicide, social isolation, loss, physical illness, easy access to lethal methods, not receiving psychiatric treatment, and cultural and religious beliefs were associated with adolescent suicides (Centers for Disease Control, 2018). The association between these risk factors and suicidal behavior has continuously been supported through ongoing empirical research (Gutierrez, Rodriguez, & Garcia, 2001; Langhinrichsen-Rohling, Arata, Bowers, O'Brien, & Morgan, 2004; Nock & Kessler, 2006; Rutter & Behrendt, 2004; Swahn & Bossart, 2007). However, research regarding risk factors for suicide-related behavior in children 13 and under has not received adequate attention. There has been insufficient focus on this younger age group and calls for further examination.

Anxiety as a risk factor

Anxiety disorders are regarded as the most common mental illness in the United States, yet only 36.9% of individuals affected receive treatment. These disorders affect 25% of children ages 13–18 (Anxiety and Depression Association of America, 2018a). Prevalence of these anxiety disorders was found to be higher in females (38%) than males (26%). A number of national organizations have begun to include anxiety disorders as essential risk factors for suicide (e.g. American Association of Suicidology, 2018; American Foundation for Suicide Prevention, 2018; National Suicide Prevention Lifeline, 2018). Individuals diagnosed with anxiety disorders have been found to be 10 times more likely to engage in suicide-related behavior than the general population (Khan, Leventhal, Khan, & Brown, 2002). Research has found that anxiety disorders were attributed to approximately 12% of suicide attempts among the United States (Bolton & Robinson, 2010).

Looking specifically at youth, the National Comorbidity Survey Adolescent Supplements (NCSA) generated data suggesting an estimated 32% of adolescents had an anxiety disorder; this included panic disorder (PD), generalized anxiety disorder (GAD), agoraphobia, specific phobia (SP), social anxiety disorder (SAD), post-traumatic stress disorder (PTSD), obsessive-compulsive disorder (OCD) and separation anxiety disorder (National Institute of Mental Health, 2018).

Anxiety can be identified as a dimensional construct, measured by the presence of an individual's state (fluctuating) and trait (stable) anxiety. Both trait and state anxiety are considered risk factors for suicidal behavior in adolescents; data also suggests that both may operate relatively independently of depression in regards to suicidality (Ohring et al., 1996). Since Mattison (1988)'s review, a sizeable number of studies have focused on this relationship between anxiety and suicide-related behavior. This relationship has been increasingly scrutinized as it has become a prevalent mental health concern. However, much of the research conducted yielded inconclusive evidence, potentially explained by methodological issues throughout the studies. For example, a review regarding anxiety's effect on suicide-related behavior amongst children and adolescents hypothesized support for the association. However, due to the little research present, the authors were unable to provide conclusive evidence to support or refute anxiety's role in suicide-related behaviors. They noted specific methodological issues throughout previous research such as: problems with how anxiety was measured (i.e. trait versus state anxiety), how depression and other variables were controlled for, as well as the temporal issue associated with anxiety (e.g., unclear if anxiety preceded the suicide-related behavior or if it was an effect of the suicide-related behavior; Hill, Castellanos, & Pettit, 2011).

Anxiety more broadly can also reflect the presence of one or more dichotomous anxiety disorder. These disorders are identified by aversive and avoidant reactions to emotional experiences (Barlow, Sauer-Zavala, Carl, Bullis, & Ellard, 2014) and, similar to suicide-related behaviors, can be conceptualized through avoidant or escape-oriented responses to emotional experiences (Baumeister, 1990; Boergers, Spirito, & Donaldson, 1998; Briere, Hodges, & Godbout, 2010; Bryan, Rudd, & Wetenberger, 2013; Shneidman, 1993). Emerging evidence suggests that anxiety-related disorders function as a risk factor for suicide-related behavior (Boden, Fergusson, & Horwood, 2007; Bolton et al., 2007; Borges, Angst, Nock, Ruscio, & Kessler, 2008; Gradus et al., 2010; Nepon, Belik, Bolton, & Sareen, 2010; Noyes, 1991; Sareen, 2011; Sareen, Cox, et al., 2005; Thibodeau, Welch, Sareen, & Asmundson, 2013; Weissman, Klerman, Markoqitz, & Ouellette, 1989; Wilcox, Storr, & Breslau, 2009). Criteria for at least one anxiety disorder were met by 70% of individuals who have had a lifetime suicide attempt (Sareen, 2011). The presence of any anxiety disorder was found to significantly increase the risk for suicidal ideation and suicide attempts. Moreover, post-traumatic stress disorder, social anxiety disorder, and panic disorder have been shown to be individually predictive of suicidal ideation (Cougle, Keough, Riccardi, & Sachs-Ericsson, 2009; Weissman et al., 1989).

Anxiety disorders and suicide-related behavior

Given the scarcity of research on the relationship between anxiety disorders and suicidal behavior in youth, we will first briefly review research findings from adult populations to serve as our theoretical foundation. Drilling down beyond anxiety more broadly and better understanding the relationship between a specific anxiety disorder and risks for suicidal behaviors may help inform future interventions.

Panic Disorder (PD) has been predominantly studied regarding it's relation to suicide, though evidence has yielded inconsistent results. A study conducted in 1989 found a strong association between suicide-related behavior and the disorder (Weissman et al., 1989) and these findings have since been replicated (Cooper, Crum & Ford, 1994; Fawcett et al., 1990; Grunhaus, Pande, Brown, & Greden, 1994; Katz, Yaseen, Mojtabai, Cohen, & Galynker, 2011; Schmidt, Woolaway-Bickel & Bates, 2005; Thibodeau et al., 2013). However, further studies have continually failed to identify PD as an individual predictor of suicide-related behavior without the presence of comorbid diagnosis or extraneous stressors (Beck, Steer, Sanderson, & Skeie, 1991; Overbeek, Rikken, Schruers, & Griez, 1998; Rudd, Dahmn, & Rajab, 1993). To date, findings do suggest PD functions as a risk factor for suicide-related behavior when coupled with co-occurring stressors (e.g., trauma exposure, depression; Albanese, Aaron, Capron, Zvolensky, & Schmidt, 2015; Nam, Kim, & Roh, 2016). Additionally, patients with PD and comorbid diagnoses are significantly more likely to have poorer prognoses and severe psycho-pathologies than individuals without PD (Grunhaus et al., 1994; Sherbourne & Wells, 1997). For example, Nam et al. (2016) found comorbid PD appears to increase the burden of the depressive symptoms in various ways (e.g., causing a more severe degree of symptoms, earlier onset, and poorer treatment courses) in patients with Major Depressive Disorder (MDD). These results also reveal comorbid PD independently increases the risk for suicide attempts among patients with MDD. Research has also found individuals with PD to struggle with psychosocial adaptation, which therefore can lead to a sense of hopelessness a known risk factor for suicide-related behavior (Nam et al., 2016). Panic attacks contributing to risk for suicidal behaviors have also been observed in adolescents (Gould et al., 1998) but not extensively studied. Very little research has emerged specifically focusing on the risk that panic disorder may have on suicidal behaviors in youth.

Social Anxiety Disorder is recognized as the second most common anxiety disorder, affecting approximately 15 million individuals in the United States. Intense anxiety and fear of being judged, evaluated negatively, or rejected in a social encounter are all characteristics of SAD. The average onset of this disorder is in teenage years and is often associated with extreme shyness in childhood, greatly impacting those diagnosed (Anxiety and Depression

Association of America, 2018a). SAD has been found to be significantly associated with high rates of suicide-related behavior, even after controlling for depression and other psychopathology (Sareen, Cox, et al., 2005).

Perceived burdensomeness (i.e., sense that one is a burden to others) and thwarted belongingness (i.e. an increased sense of alienation from others) have both been actively associated with suicide-related behavior (Van Orden, Cukrowicz, Witte, & Joiner, 2012) and can be present in an individual with SAD. Both of these risk factors have been highlighted in the Interpersonal-Psychological Theory of Suicide (Joiner, 2005). Thwarted belongingness is directly linked to a common characteristic of SAD: social avoidance. Lower rates of self-esteem are found amongst individuals with SAD and can lead to a sense of being undeserving of others' support, potentially contributing to this perception that he or she is a burden (Ritter, Ertel, Beil, Steffens, & Stangier, 2013; Van Orden et al., 2012). A recent study examining the relationship between SAD and these two risk factors for suicide-related behavior found social anxiety to be significantly related to thwarted belonging-ingness as well as perceived burdensomeness. This was found even after for controlling for co-occurring variables (i.e. depression, demographic information, and substance-use; Bucker, Lemke, Jeffies, & Shah, 2017).

Findings indicate socially anxious adults are 73% more likely to remain single and live alone compared to depressed individuals (Teo, Lerrigo, & Rogers, 2013). Due to the symptoms associated with SAD causing interference with daily functioning (i.e. ability to attend a job interview, occupational performance, social situations, maintain relationships or friendships), social avoidance is highly prevalent in this disorder (Anxiety and Depression Association of America, 2018b). By determining that interpersonal impairment among socially anxious individuals increases their vulnerability to suicidal ideation, findings support the relationship between SAD and suicide-related behavior (Bucker et al., 2017). Unfortunately, less than 5% of people diagnosed with SAD seek treatment in the year following the initial onset. In addition to this, a third of individuals suffering from SAD symptoms do not report symptoms or seek treatment for 10 or more years (Anxiety and Depression Association of America, 2018b). Not only does this population often remain undiagnosed and therefore untreated (Grant et al., 2005), they are suffering from symptoms that can be considered risk factors for suicide-related behavior.

SAD has been found to increase the risk for suicide-related behavior specifically amongst the adolescent population. Research indicates social anxiety symptoms are concurrently associated with suicide-related behavior specifically among adolescents (Nelson et al., 2000; Valentiner, Gutierrez, & Blacker, 2002). Through the examination of clinically referred young adolescents, Gallagher, Prinstein, Simon, and Spirito (2014) predicted suicidal ideation 18 months post-baseline, after controlling for other psychiatric diagnoses (e.g., depression). Similar to previous studies, these findings indicate suicide-related behavior in the adolescent population may persist in adulthood ages. As adolescence is a defining age with individuals developing social relationships, the social withdrawal or deficit associated with SAD may interfere with this developmental period. This could lead to increased isolation and hopelessness, two known risk factors for suicide-related behavior. The results demonstrate that loneliness significantly mediated this variance, exhibited between suicidal ideation at baseline compared to 18 months post-baseline (Gallagher et al., 2014). Consistent with previous literature proposing the link between loneliness and increased suicidality (Schnika, Van Dulmen, Bossarte, & Swahn, 2012), these findings further support SAD as a risk factor for suicide-related behavior.

Generalized Anxiety Disorder is most frequently studied in relation to its comorbidity with mood disorders, rather than as a stand-alone risk factor for suicidality. GAD affects approximately 3% of the United States' population. This anxiety disorder is marked by persistent and excessive worry about a variety of facets in life (e.g., health, family, work) often leading one to anticipate disaster as it is extremely difficult to curb the worry (Anxiety and Depression Association of American, 2018c). GAD is consistently associated with various somatic symptoms, sleep disorders and chronic pain conditions as well as being frequently comorbid with PD, SAD, specific phobia (SP), and PTSD (Nutt, Argyropoulos, Hood, & Potokar, 2006). As mentioned above, comorbidity between GAD and mood and MDD is often found (Judd et al., 2007; Ninan, 2001). These high rates of comorbidity elevate the hardship and affect GAD has on the individuals diagnosed. This leads to the individual's further impairment, increased severity of symptoms as well as frequent inaccurate diagnoses and treatment approaches (Nutt et al., 2006). Research suggests higher levels of suicidality among individuals with GAD compared to those with univariate symptoms of depression (Zimmerman & Chelminski, 2003).

Similar to adult findings, there has been some research to support GAD, particularly in the context of depression, as a risk factor for suicidal behaviors in adolescents as well (e.g., Foley, Goldston, Costello, & Angold, 2006; Strauss et al., 2000). It may be that the comorbidity between GAD and depression highlights the transdiagnostic process of rumination as a risk factor for suicidal behaviors. While research in this area is emerging for children and adolescents, it warrants further understanding.

OCD and suicide-related behavior

Obsessive-Compulsive Disorder (OCD) is a disorder which often includes anxiety as a prominent feature. OCD has emerged in recent years as a disorder also linked to suicidality. It is characterized by intrusive and persistent anxiety-producing thoughts (obsessions) and repetitive behaviors in order to control these thoughts (compulsions). These compulsions often are manifested in increasingly time-consuming rituals, conducted in order to ease the distress caused by these intrusive obsessive thoughts (American Psychiatric Association, 2013). OCD is regarded as a major mental health condition, ranked within the top 10 most disabling conditions globally, characterized by a significant decline in an individual's functioning (Murray & Lopez, 1996). The disorder is distinguished by severe distress, high levels of disability, and overall disruption of an individual's social and occupational functioning (Crino, Slade, & Andrews, 2005; Vaele & Roberts, 2014).

The largest international evaluation of OCD comorbidity indicated suicidal ideation among this population occurred frequently, finding that previous suicide attempts were also prevalent (Brakoulias et al., 2017). Earlier studies were able to adjust for comorbidity and support OCD as an independent predictor of suicide risk (De la Cruz et al., 2016). Findings indicate that 10–27% of those suffering from OCD may attempt suicide at least once in their lifetime (Hollander et al., 2014; Kamath, Reddy, & Kandavel, 2007; Torres et al., 2007) and 41–97% has been found to endorse suicidal thoughts (Gupta, Avasthi, Grover, & Singh, 2014; Khosravani, Zoleikha, Ardakani, & Ardestani, 2017; Torres et al., 2007, 2013). Specifically, obsessions have been strongly associated with suicide-related behavior when compared to compulsions, suggesting that these obsessions operate as a mechanism linking the disorder to suicidality (Dell'Osso et al., 2012; Philips et al., 2007). These obsessions (i.e. intrusive thoughts, images or impulses) generate severe anxiety among the individuals affected (American Psychiatric Association, 2017). Experiencing intrusive, unacceptable thoughts have been found to cause increased shame and fear, coupled with decreased social acceptance than those void of these thoughts (Dell'Osso et al., 2012). Known risk factors for suicide-related behavior, including hopelessness and a past history of suicidality, have been found to be strongly associated with suicidality among individuals with OCD (O'Connor & Nock, 2014). Current evidence detailing the association between OCD and suicide-related behavior has yielded inconclusive results, often due to unsystematic methodology. However, a recent meta-analysis revealed a moderate to significant association between suicidality and OCD. The study identified potential mechanisms involved in the relationship between OCD and suicide-related behavior, including, comorbid psychopathology, the severity of anxiety and depressive symptoms, hopelessness, as well as a history of suicidality. It was found that the comorbidity of psychopathology (primarily depression, bipolar disorder, and psychoses) did increase the likelihood of suicide-related behavior in individuals with OCD (Angelakis, Gooding, Tarrier, & Panagioti, 2015). While the study did not account for comorbid disorders, the overall severity of OCD symptoms has been found to have a significant contribution to suicide-related behavior (Philips et al., 2007; Sareen, Cox, et al., 2005). Very little research has been conducted to examine the potential risk of OCD and suicidal behavior in children and adolescents. Given the growing evidence in adult literature, exploring this relationship for youth is an important next step to consider.

PTSD & suicide-related behavior

Post-traumatic stress disorder is also a specific disorder where anxiety can potentially be a prominent feature. Research has found PTSD to be the specific disorder with the most empirical support as a unique predictor of suicide-related behavior (e.g., Sareen, Houlahan, et al., 2005). PTSD is a disorder one is susceptible to developing following a traumatic life event. This event can vary in nature (e.g., the loss of a loved one, physical or sexual trauma, near-death experience, etc.) and can develop in an ongoing chronic manner or in a short-term acute way. Typical symptoms associated with PTSD include: re-experiencing (e.g., flashbacks of the trauma), avoidance (e.g., averting thoughts and feelings related to the trauma), arousal and/or activity (e.g., becoming easily startled or angered), and cognitive and/or mood symptoms (e.g., distorted feelings, loss of interest, difficulty remembering trauma). The disorder is recognized by the individual's inability to function daily due to these pervasive symptoms stemming from said traumatic event (National Institute of Mental Health, 2018). Of note, hyperarousal and sleep deprivation are both commonly seen in individuals suffering from PTSD, both of which may be specifically important regarding the risk for suicide-related behavior (Sareen, Houlahan, Cox, & Asmundson, 2005).

Through the use of a nationally representative sample of United States residents ages 15–54, the National Comorbidity Survey found individuals suffering from PTSD were 6 times more likely to attempt suicide than demographically compared controls (Kessler, Borges, & Walters, 1999). PTSD has consistently been linked to suicide-related behavior even after controlling for depressive symptoms (Davidson, Hughes, Blazer, & George, 1991). However, research had yielded inconsistent results as to if this link is significant (Breslau, Lucia, & Alvarado, 2006; Storr, Ialongo, Anthony, & Breslau, 2007). Wilcox et al. (2009) conducted a study to determine if PTSD was directly and independently related to suicide-related behavior or if the trauma individuals experienced was the risk factor playing a role. This study generated results linking individuals with PTSD to a later suicide attempt of which was sustained after adjusting for other established risk factors (e.g., sex, pre-existing depression). Yet, this link was not maintained among individuals solely exposed to the trauma of who did not meet criteria for a PTSD diagnosis. These results therefore indicate the increased risk for suicide-related behavior is derived from the anxiety disorder rather than the traumatic event itself. The results did not fluctuate dependent upon the type of traumatic event each individual experienced (e.g., assaultive violence, car accident, a natural disaster, witnessing homicide or serious injury, learning of loved one's assault). While this study did pose limitations (e.g., recall bias, small sample size), it was able to utilize a teenage population, bolstering the limited research on this population (Wilcox et al., 2009).

Comorbidity & demographics

Anxiety disorders are found to be comorbid among themselves as well as with other disorders. Kendall et al. (2010) studied youth ages 7–17, finding 55% of the participants met criteria for one or more disorders in addition to one of the three anxiety disorders of focus (Separation Anxiety Disorder, Generalized Anxiety Disorder, and Social Phobia). Left untreated, anxiety disorders in children can predict anxiety disorders and depression in adulthood (Ferdinand, Verhulst, & Wiznitzer, 1995; Kendall, Safford, Flannery-Schroeder, & Webb, 2004; Pine, Cohen, & Gurley, 1998). While anxiety has been inconsistently supported as a risk factor for suicide-related behavior, it is frequently associated with other known risk factors (i.e. depression, social isolation, hopelessness; Abreu et al., 2018).

Depression is the most common psychiatric disorder in people who die by suicide; this has found to be a risk factor for suicide-related behavior and has been thoroughly examined as such (Hawton et al., 2013). While this research has yielded clinically relevant results, the focus has been narrow by primarily investigating common risk factors such as depression. However, less empirical consideration has been given to the relationship between suicide-related behavior and other forms of psychopathology, such as anxiety disorders (Norton, Temple, & Pettit, 2008). The relationship between depression and anxiety has been heavily studied and viewed through three conceptual models: anxiety and depression as categorical disorders with distinct boundaries; anxiety and depression as an overlapping continuum; and as a mixed disorder that differs from the single forms of these disorders (Shores et al., 1992).

Given that depression has been significantly linked to suicide-related behavior, and there is a high comorbidity rate between depression and anxiety, the role of anxiety may also contribute as a risk factor. This high comorbidity is a prominent feature that complicates the examination of anxiety as a risk factor associated with suicide-related behavior (e.g., Brown, Campbell, Lehman, Gisham, & Mancill, 2001). There has been debate as to if anxiety is an artifact of depression or if it operates independently regarding its effect on suicide-related behavior. As this question has emerged, research has attempted to control for depression when examining anxiety's association with suicide-related behavior (e.g., Bucker et al., 2017; Norton et al., 2008; Ohring et al., 1996). In doing so, findings continue to suggest a significant association between anxiety and suicidality, independent of depression (Sareen, Cox, et al., 2005). Norton et al. (2008) also found depression and anxiety have a unique interactive effect on suicidality, suggesting an elevation of both may account for additional risk. Importantly, suicidal ideation is found to be six times more likely among individuals diagnosed with two or more anxiety disorders compared to individuals without an anxiety disorder (Boden et al., 2007).

Additionally, Khosravani et al. (2017) found a strong association between childhood trauma (e.g., sexual abuse) and suicide-related behavior among individuals (ages 15–80) with OCD. The study found 97% of those diagnosed with OCD who also experienced childhood trauma were found to have current suicidal ideation; revealing higher rates of depression, suicidal ideation, and anxiety than the controls. Similarly, previous findings suggest childhood sexual abuse inflicted, comorbid with OCD symptoms, is related to the higher prevalence of suicide attempts (46%) than abuse victims without OCD (28%; Peles, Schrieber, & Adleson, 2009).

There has also been research to suggest important sociodemographic information need to be considered both in suicidal behaviors in general and the relationship between risk factors and suicidal behaviors. White individuals were found to commit suicide most frequently, followed by American Indians and Alaska Natives. Adult females reported a suicide attempt 1.2 times as often as males (American Foundation for Suicide Prevention, 2018). While females were found to attempt suicide significantly more often than males, males have been found to complete suicide significantly more often. This was determined through the examination of suicide-related behavior and how it acts as a function among both genders and across all cultural groups (Langhinrichsen-Rohling, Friend, & Powell, 2009). Revealing important differences between the relationships among various anxiety disorders and suicide-related behavior, findings indicate noteworthy gender differences. Among the adult population, GAD, SAD, PTSD, and PD have been found to predict suicidal ideation among women; PTSD was the only disorder predictive of suicidal ideation among men (Cougle et al., 2009).

Specific considerations for youth

Anxiety disorders in childhood and adolescence are not only prevalent, but can cause significant psychosocial impairment (Bernstien & Borchardt, 1991; Bernstien, Borchardt, & Perwien, 1996; Ginsburg, La Greca, & Silverman, 1998). This can be evidenced by a child's decrease in daily functioning as a result of said disorder. For example, research has suggested that children with anxiety disorders are more likely to have a poor relationship with peers as well as impaired perceived self-competence (i.e. indicated by social isolation as a result of behavioral avoidance; Bowen, Offord, & Boyle, 1990; Olatunji et al., 2007). The impact anxiety disorders have on this population raises concerns for the child's risk for maladaptive behaviors (e.g., negative self-talk), that could then lead to suicide-related behavior (Kendall et al., 2010).

The literature predominantly focuses on the adult population regarding the role anxiety disorders play as a risk factor for suicide-related behavior. The diagnoses, symptoms, and disorders fortunately have been widely studied among the adult population. However, our review highlights the paucity of literature focusing on risk factors associated with suicide-related behavior as well as the role anxiety disorders potentially play in youth. Through reviewing the existing literature, it is clear how narrow the scope has been to date. This has been a recurring phenomenon as studying suicide-related behavior among child and adolescents is challenging. Limitations naturally accompany this age group given the taboo nature of admitting that children and teens experience and engage in suicidal behaviors. Unique barriers in conducting research with children in the context of suicidal behaviors include challenges in recruitment, consent, and the discomfort adults experience in acknowledging that children experience something as discomforting as suicidal ideation, let alone intent and follow through.

Given the areas identified in adult literature highlighting the link between anxiety disorders to suicide-related behavior among adults, it is crucial to further this examination among children and adolescents. As noted previously, suicide is the second leading cause of death among ages 10–34 (Centers for Disease Control, 2018). Despite research-supporting suicide as a common concern among this population, there is strikingly insufficient research focusing categorically on the child and adolescent ages. Very little research has examined the risk these disorders pose among younger populations, despite findings supporting the link among adult populations. While research among adult populations can potentially be generalized to younger ages, specific focus on children and adolescents is crucial. As support continues to emerge regarding anxiety as a risk factor for suicide-related behavior, suggesting that the presence of "any anxiety disorder" increases risk in the general population, examination of this among specific populations (e.g., children) is warranted (Boden et al., 2007; Sareen, Cox, et al., 2005).

Implications for practice

While highlighting gaps in existing literature may be relatively straightforward, the more pressing questions center on how we move forward as a field to address these gaps. As mentioned above, conducting research with youth has unique barriers; but that should not deter researchers from pursuing a more nuanced understanding of suicidal behavior in children. Indeed, given the data suggesting that suicidal behaviors in children and adolescents are growing, the need for rigorous research within this domain needs to be addressed. Given there are potential links between specific anxiety disorders and risk for suicidal behaviors, researchers should consider exploring and reporting on suicidal behaviors within research on anxiety in children and adolescents. An additional consideration is to continue to focus efforts on more transdiagnostic processes that may contribute to suicidal behaviors in youth, beyond focusing on the psychopathology of depression. The research on social anxiety and the role of perceived burdensomeness and thwarted belongingness is an excellent example of expanding comorbidity research to focus on more transdiagnostic processes. Providing empirical support for these processes also has the potential to lead to developing more tailored interventions with far-reaching positive outcomes.

In regards to clinical practice, anxiety disorders emerge as diagnoses that should be taken seriously. While this point may seem elementary, anxiety disorders are not often thought of within the context of suicidal risk, particularly when compared to mood disorders, and especially in the context of working with children and adolescents. For the individual clinician, risk assessments should be conducted for all intakes, regardless of presenting problem. Many clinicians are trained to inquire about suicidal thoughts/ behaviors in the context of depressive symptoms, but less likely to be considered when discussing anxiety symptoms.

Given the growing findings surrounding the role, anxiety can play in suicidal ideation for children/adolescents, the need to evolve our training of mental health practitioners should be considered. Trainings to consider fall into two categories, trainings tailored to increase the comfort level of assessing for suicidal ideation/behaviors specifically in children/adolescents and training that broadens the understanding of risk factors for suicidal ideation/behaviors beyond depression.

Of note, a number of suicide prevention programs are evolving that target school communities. The need for these programs has been recognized and many communities are working to address these issues in schools. However, these programs are more likely to target discussions around depression symptoms (e.g., Rice, & Sher 2015); while research is immerging to support multiple pathways to suicide in children and adolescents (e.g., impulsivity; Sheftall et al., 2016). Furthermore, while schools are working to implement suicide prevention programs to support their students, some research has shown that widely used programs specifically targeting suicide prevention may not be evidence-based (e.g., Cooper, Clements, & Holt, 2011; Wei, Kutcher, & LeBlanc, 2015). It is recommended that if schools are considering channeling resources into a prevention program, one that is evidence-based and targeting underlying processes (e.g., anxiety, depression) that contribute to suicidal ideation/behaviors are worth considering.

In addition to schools, pediatricians are often the first line of defense in regards to child mental health care. Parents are more likely to take their child to a pediatrician first if they have any concerns, before trying to navigate the mental health system. Advancing the education of pediatricians to consider anxiety as a risk factor for suicidality will in turn provide parents with important information. Increasing trainings on risk assessments for professionals is an important avenue to consider. Outdated theories around talking about suicide with youth increasing their risk have been debunked but may still be a fear held by professionals (Pettit, Buitron & Green, 2018).

Overall, anxiety as a risk factor for suicidal behavior in youth continues to be an area for further study. This need is present within research, but clinicians should also consider anxiety as an avenue worth exploring in the service of understanding and treating suicidal behaviors in youth.

Disclosure statement

No potential conflict of interest was reported by the authors.

References

Abreu, L. N., Oquendo, M. A., Burke, A., Grunebaum, M. F., Sher, L., Sullivan, G. M., … Lafer, B. (2018). Are comorbid anxiety disorders a risk factor for suicide attempts in patients with mood disorders? A two-year prospective study. *European Psychiatry*, *47*, 19–24. doi:10.1016/j.eurpsy.2017.09.005

Albanese, B. J., Aaron, M. N., Capron, D. W., Zvolensky, M. J., & Schmidt, N. B. (2015). Panic symptoms and elevated suicidal ideation and behaviors among trauma exposed individuals: Moderating effects of post-traumatic stress disorder. *Comprehensive Psychiatry*, *61*, 42–48. doi:10.1016/j.comppsych.2015.05.006

Alonso, P., Segala, C., Real, E., Pertusa, A., Labad, J., Jimenez-Murcia, S., … & Menchón, J. M. (2010). Suicide in patients treated for obsessive-compulsive disorder: A prospective follow-up study. *Journal of Affective Disorders*, *144*, 300–308. doi:10.1016/j.jad.2009.12.001

American Association of Suicidology (2018). Facts and Statistics, National Suicide Statistics. Retrieved from June 15, 2018. https://www.suicidology.org/resources/facts-statistics

American Foundation for Suicide Prevention, (2015). Suicide statistics. Retrieved from October 16, 2018. https://afsp.org/aboutsuicide/suicide-statistics/.

American Foundation for Suicide Prevention. (2018). *About suicide – Suicide statistics*. Retrieved from https://afsp.org/about-suicide/suicide-statistics/

American Psychiatric Association, (2013). *Obsessive-Compulsive Disorder – What is Obsessive-Compulsive Disorder?* Retrieved from October 16, 2018. https://www.psychiatry.org/patients-families/ocd/what-is-obsessive-compulsive-disorder

American Psychiatric Associaton. (2017). *Obsessive-Compulsive Disorder – What is Obsessive-Compulsive Disorder?* Retrieved from https://www.psychiatry.org/patients-families/ocd/what isobsessive-compulsive-disorder.

Angelakis, I., Gooding, P., Tarrier, N., & Panagioti, M. (2015). Suicidality in obsessive compulsive disorder (OCD): A systematic review and meta-analysis. *Clinical Psychology Review*, *39*, 1–15. doi:10.1016/j.cpr.2015.03.002

Anxiety and Depression Association of America. (2018a). *Facts and statistics*. Retrieved from https://adaa.org/about-adaa/press-room/facts-statistics

Anxiety and Depression Association of America. (2018b). *Understanding the facts – Social anxiety disorder*. Retrieved from https://adaa.org/understanding- anxiety/social-anxiety-disorder

Anxiety and Depression Association of America. (2018c). *Generalized Anxiety Disorder (GAD) – Understanding GAD and the symptoms*. Retrieved from https://adaa.org/under standing-anxiety/generalized-anxiety-disorder-gad

Balici, V., & Sevincok, L. (2010). Suicidal ideation in patients with obsessive-compulsive disorder. *Psychiatry Research, 175*, 104–108. doi:10.1016/j.psychres.2009.03.012

Barlow, D. H., Sauer-Zavala, S., Carl, J. R., Bullis, J. R., & Ellard, K. K. (2014). The nature, diagnosis, and treatment of neuroticism. *Clinical Psychological Science, 2*(3), 344–365.

Baumeister, R. F. (1990). Suicide as escape from self. *Psychological Review, 97*(1), 90–113. doi:10.1037/0033-295X.97.1.90

Beck, A. T., Steer, R. A., Sanderson, W. C., & Skeie, T. M. (1991). Panic disorder and suicidal ideation and behavior: Discrepant findings in psychiatric outpatients. *American Journal of Psychiatry, 148*(9), 1195–1199.

Bernstien, G. A., & Borchardt, C. M. (1991). Anxiety disorders of childhood and adolescence: A critical review. *Journal of American Academy of Child Adolescent Psychiatry, 30*(4), 519–532.

Bernstien, G. A., Borchardt, C. M., & Perwien, B. A. (1996). Anxiety disorders in children and adolescents: A review of the past 10 years. *Journal of the American Academy of Child & Adolescent Psychiatry, 35*(9), 1110–1119. doi:10.1097/00004583-199609000-00008

Boden, J. M., Fergusson, D. M., & Horwood, J. (2007). Anxiety disorders and suicidal behaviours in adolescence and young adulthood: Findings from a longitudinal study. *Psychological Medicine, 37*(3), 431–440. doi:10.1017/S0033291706009147

Bodzy, M. E., Barreto, S. J., Swenson, L. P., Liguori, G., & Costea, G. (2016). Self-reported psychopathology, trauma symptoms, and emotion coping among child suicide attempters and ideators: An exploratory study of young children. *Archives of Suicide Research, 20*(2), 160–175.

Boergers, J., Spirito, A., & Donaldson, D. (1998). Reasons for adolescent suicide attempts: Associations with psychological functioning. *Journal of the American Academy of Child & Adolescent Psychiatry, 37*(12), 1287–1293. doi:10.1097/00004583-199812000-00012

Bolton, J. M., Cox, B. J., Afifi, T. O., Enns, M. W., Bienvenu, O. J., & Sareen, J. (2007). Anxiety disorders and risk for suicide attempts: Findings from the Baltimore epidemiologic catchment area follow-up study. *Journal of Depression and Anxiety, 25*(6), 447–481.

Bolton, J. M., & Robinson, J. (2010). Population-attributable fractions of Axis I and Axis II mental disorders for suicide attempts: Findings from a representative sample of the adult, noninstitutionalized US population. *American Journal of Public Health, 100*, 2473–2480. doi:10.2105/AJPH.2010.192252

Borges, G., Angst, J., Nock, M. K., Ruscio, A. M., & Kessler, R. (2008). Risk factors for the incidence of suicide-related outcomes: A 10-year follow-up study using the national comorbidity surveys. *Journal of Affective Disorders, 105*(1–3), 25–33. doi:10.1016/j. jad.2007.01.036

Bowen, R. C., Offord, D. R., & Boyle, M. H. (1990). The prevalence of overanxious disorder and separation anxiety disorder: Results from the Ontario child health study. *Child and Adolescent Psychiatry, 29*(5), 753–758. doi:10.1097/00004583-199009000-00013

Brakoulias, V., Starcevic, V., Belloch, A., Brown, C., Ferrao, Y. A., Fontenelle, L. F., ... Viswasam, K. (2017). Comorbidity, age of onset and suicidality in obsessive-compulsive disorder (OCD): An international collaboration. *Comprehensive Psychiatry, 76*, 79–86. doi:10.1016/j.comppsych.2017.04.002

Breslau, N., Lucia, V. C., & Alvarado, G. F. (2006). Intelligence and other predisposing factors in exposure to trauma and posttraumatic stress disorder: A follow-up study at age 17 years. *Archives of General Psychiatry*, *63*(11), 1238–1245. doi:10.1001/archpsyc.63.11.1238

Briere, J., Hodges, M., & Godbout, N. (2010). Traumatic stress, affect dysregulation, and dysfunctional avoidance: A structural equation model. *Journal of Traumatic Stress*, *23*(6), 767–774. doi:10.1002/jts.20578

Brodsky, B. S., Oquendo, M., Ellis, S. P., Haas, G. L., Malone, K. M., & Mann, J. J. (2001). The relationship of childhood abuse to impulsivity and suicidal behavior in adults with major depression. *The American Journal of Psychiatry*, *158*(11), 1871–1877. doi:10.1176/appi. ajp.158.11.1871

Brown, T. A., Campbell, L. A., Lehman, C. L., Gisham, J. R., & Mancill, R. B. (2001). Current and lifetime comorbidity of the DSM-IV anxiety and mood disorders in a large clinical sample. *Journal of Abnormal Psychology*, *110*(4), 585–599. doi:10.1037/0021-843X.110.4.585

Bryan, C. J., Rudd, M. D., & Wetenberger, E. (2013). Reasons for suicide attempts in a clinical sample of active duty soldiers. *Journal of Affective Disorders*, *144*, 148–152. doi:10.1016/j. jad.2012.06.030

Bucker, J. D., Lemke, A. W., Jeffies, E. R., & Shah, S. M. (2017). Social anxiety and suicidal ideation: Test of the utility of the interpersonal psychological theory of suicide. *Journal of Anxiety Disorders*, *45*, 60–63. doi:10.1016/j.janxdis.2016.11.010

Cavanagh, J. T., Carson, A. J., Sharpe, M., & Lawrie, S. M. (2003). Psychological autopsy studies of suicide: A systematic review. *Psychological Medicine*, *33*, 395–405. doi:10.1017/S0033291702006943

Centers for Disease Control. (2018). *Youth risk behavior surveillance – United States, surveillance summaries, MMWR, 59*. Retrieved from https://www.cdc.gov/violenceprevention/suicide/statistics/index.html

Cooper, G. D., Clements, P. T., & Holt, K. (2011). A review and application of suicide prevention programs in high school settings. *Issues in Mental Health Nursing*, *32*, 696–702. doi:10.3109/01612840.2011.576326

Cooper-Patrick, L., Crum, R. M., & Ford, D. E. (1994). Identifying suicidal ideation in general medical patients. *JAMA*, *272*(2), 1757–1762.

Cougle, J. R., Keough, M. E., Riccardi, C. J., & Sachs-Ericsson, N. (2009). Anxiety disorders and suicidality in the national comorbidity survey-replication. *Journal of Psychiatric Research*, *43*, 825–829. doi:10.1016/j.jpsychires.2008.12.004

Crino, R., Slade, T., & Andrews, G. (2005). The changing prevalence and severity of obsessive-compulsive disorder criteria from DSM-III to DSM-I. *American Journal of Psychiatry*, *162*, 876–992. doi:10.1176/appi.ajp.162.5.876

Davidson, J. R., Hughes, D., Blazer, D. G., & George, L. K. (1991). Post-traumatic stress disorder in the community: An epidemiological study. *Psychological Medicine*, *21*(3), 713–721. doi:10.1017/S0033291700022352

De la Cruz, L. F., Rydell, M., Runeson, B., O'nofrio, B., Brander, G., Ruck, C., ... & Mataix-Cols, D. (2016). Suicide in obsessive-compulsive disorder: A population-based study of 36,788 Swedish patients. *Molecular Psychiatry*, *22*, 1626.

Dell'Osso, L., Casu, G., Carlini, M., Conversano, C., Gremigni, P., & Carmassi, C. (2012). Sexual obsessions and suicidal behaviors in patients with mood disorders, panic disorder, and schizophrenia. *Annals of General Psychiatry*, *11*, 27. doi:10.1186/1744-859X-11-27

Fawcett, J., Scheftner, W. A., Fogg, L., Clark, D. C., Young, M. A., Hedeker, D., Gibbons, R. (1990). Time-related predictors of suicide in major affective disorder. *American Journal of Psychiatry*, *147*(9), 1189–1194.

Ferdinand, R. F., Verhulst, F. C., & Wiznitzer, M. (1995). Continuity and change of self-reported problem behaviors and adolescence into young adulthood. *Child and Adolescent Psychiatry, 24*(5), 680–690. doi:10.1097/00004583-199505000-00020

Foley, D. L., Goldston, D. B., Costello, J., & Angold, A. (2006). Proximal psychiatric risk factors for suicidality in youth. *Archives of General Psychiatry, 63*, 1017–1024. doi:10.1001/archpsyc.63.9.1017

Gallagher, M., Prinstein, M. J., Simon, V., & Spirito, A. (2014). Social anxiety symptoms and suicidal ideation in a clinical sample of early adolescents: Examining loneliness and social support as longitudinal mediators. *Journal of Abnormal Clinical Psychology, 42*, 871–883. doi:10.1007/s10802-013-9844-7

Ginsburg, G. S., La Greca, A. M., & Silverman, W. K. (1998). Social anxiety in children with anxiety disorders: Relation with social and emotional functioning. *Journal of Abnormal Child Psychology, 26*(3), 175–185. doi:10.1023/A:1022668101048

Goodwin, D. W., Guze, S. B., & Robings, E. (1969). Follow-up studies in obsessional neurosis. *Archives of General Psychiatry, 20*, 182–187. doi:10.1001/archpsyc.1969.01740140054006

Gould, M. S., King, R., Greenwald, S., Fisher, P., Schwab-Stone, M., Kramer, R., … Shaffer, D. (1998). Psychopathology associated with suicidal ideation and attempts among children and adolescents. *Journal of American Academy of Child and Adolescent Psychiatry, 37*(9), 915–923. doi:10.1097/00004583-199809000-00011

Gradus, J. L., Qin, P., Lincoln, A. K., Miller, M., Lawler, E., Sorensen, H. T., & Lash, T. L. (2010). Post-traumatic stress disorder and completed suicide. *American Journal of Epidemiology, 171*(6), 721–727. doi:10.1093/aje/kwp456

Grant, B. F., Hasin, D. S., Blanco, C., Stinson, F. S., Chou, S. P., Goldstein, R. B., & Huang, B. (2005). The epidemiology of social anxiety disorder in the United States: Results from the national epidemiologic survey on alcohol and related conditions. *Journal of Clinical Psychiatry, 66*(1), 1351–1361.

Grunhaus, L., Pande, A. C., Brown, M. B., & Greden, J. F. (1994). Clinical characteristics of patients with concurrent major depressive disorder and panic disorder. *American Journal of Psychiatry, 151*, 541–546. doi:10.1176/ajp.151.4.541

Gupta, G., Avasthi, A., Grover, S., & Singh, S. M. (2014). Factors associated with suicidal ideations and suicidal attempts in patients with obsessive compulsive disorder. *Asian Journal of Psychiatry, 12*, 140–146. doi:10.1016/j.ajp.2014.09.004

Gutierrez, P. M., Rodriguez, P. J., & Garcia, P. (2001). Suicide risk factors for young adults: Testing a model across ethnicities. *Journal of Death Studies, 25*(4), 319–340. doi:10.1080/07481180151143088

Hawton, K., Comabella, C. C., Haw, C., & Saunders, K. (2013). Risk factors for suicide in individuals with depression: A systematic review. *Journal of Affective Disorders, 147*, 17–28. doi:10.1016/j.jad.2013.01.004

Hill, R., Castellanos, D., & Pettit, J. W. (2011). Suicide-related behaviors and anxiety in children and adolescents: A review. *Clinical Psychology Review, 31*, 1133–1144. doi:10.1016/j.cpr.2011.07.008

Hollander, E., Greenwald, S., Neville, D., Johnson, J., Hornig, C. D., & Weissman, M. M. (2014). Uncomplicated and comorbid obsessive-compulsive disorder in an epidemiologic sample. *CNS Spectrums, 3*, 10–18. doi:10.1017/S1092852900007148

Joiner, T. E., Jr. (2005). *Why people die by suicide*. Cambridge, MA, US: Harvard University Press.

Judd, L. L., Kessler, R. C., Paulus, M. P., Zeller, P. V., Wittchen, H. U., & Kunovac, J. L. (2007). Comorbidity as a fundamental feature of generalized anxiety disorders: Results from the National Comorbidity Study (NCS). *Acta Psychiatricia Scandinavica*, *98*(393), 6–11. doi:10.1111/j.1600-0447.1998.tb05960.x

Kamath, P., Reddy, Y. C. J., & Kandavel, T. (2007). Suicidal behavior in obsessive-compulsive disorder. *Journal of Clinical Psychiatry*, *68*, 1741–1750. doi:10.4088/JCP.v68n1114

Katz, C., Yaseen, Z. S., Mojtabai, R., Cohen, L. J., & Galynker, I. I. (2011). Panic as an independent risk factor for suicide attempt in depressive illness: Findings from the National Epidemiological Survey on Alcohol Related Conditions (NESARC). *Journal of Clinical Psychiatry*, *72*, 1628–1635. doi:10.4088/JCP.09m05440blu

Kendall, P. C., Compton, S. N., Walkup, J. T., Brimaher, B., Albano, A. M., Sherrill, J., ... Piacentini, J. (2010). Clinical characteristics of anxiety disordered youth. *Journal of Anxiety Disorders*, *24*(3), 360–365. doi:10.1016/j.janxdis.2010.01.009

Kendall, P. C., Safford, S., Flannery-Schroeder, E., & Webb, A. (2004). Child anxiety treatment: Outcomes in adolescence and impact on substance use and depression at 7.4-year follow-up. *Journal of Consulting and Clinical Psychology*, *72*(2), 276–287. doi:10.1037/0022-006X.72.2.276

Kessler, R. C., Borges, G., & Walters, E. E. (1999). Prevalence of the risk factors for lifetime suicide attempts in the national comorbidity survey. *Archives of General Psychiatry*, *56*(7), 617–626.

Khan, A., Leventhal, R. M., Khan, S., & Brown, W. A. (2002). Suicide risk in patients with anxiety disorders: A meta-analysis of the FDA database. *Journal of Affective Disorders*, *68*, 83–190. doi:10.1016/S0165-0327(01)00354-8

Khosravani, V., Zoleikha, K., Ardakani, R. J., & Ardestani, M. S. (2017). The relation of childhood trauma to suicide ideation in patients suffering from obsessive-compulsive disorder with lifetime suicide attempts. *Psychiatry Research*, *255*, 139–145. doi:10.1016/j.psychres.2017.05.032

Langhrinrichsen-Rohling, J., Arata, C., Bowers, D., O'Brien, N., & Morgan, A. (2004). Suicidal behavior, negative affect, gender, and self-reported delinquency in college students. *Suicide and Life- Threatening Behavior*, *34*(3), 255–266.

Langhrinrichsen-Rohling, J., Friend, J., & Powell, A. (2009). Adolescent suicide, gender, and culture: A rate and risk factor analysis. *Aggression and Violent Behavior*, *14*, 402–414.

Malone, K. M., Haas, G. L., Sweeney, J. A., & Mann, J. J. (1995). Major depression and the risk of attempted suicide. *Journal of Affective Disorders*, *35*(3), 173–185. doi:10.1016/0165-0327(95)00015-F

Mattison, R. E. (1988). Suicide and other consequences of childhood and adolescent anxiety disorders. *The Journal of Clinical Psychiatry*, *49*(10), 9–11.

Murray, C., & Lopez, A. (1996). *Global health statistics: A compendium of incidence, prevalence and mortality estimates over 2000 conditions.* Cambridge, MA: Harvard University Press.

Nam, Y., Kim, C. H., & Roh, D. (2016). Comorbid panic disorder as an independent risk factor for suicide attempts in depressed outpatients. *Comprehensive Psychiatry*, *67*, 13–18. doi:10.1016/j.comppsych.2016.02.011

National Institute of Mental Health. (2018). *Mental health information – Statistics.* Retrieved from https://www.nimh.nih.gov/health/statistics/suicide.shtml

National Suicide Prevention Lifeline. (2018). *We can all prevent suicide – Know the risk factors.* Retrieved from https://suicidepreventionlifeline.org/how-we-can- all-prevent-suicide/

Nelson, E. C., Grant, J. D., Bucholz, K. K., Glowinski, A., Madden, P. A. F., Reich, W., & Heath, A. C. (2000). Social phobia in a population-based female adolescent twin sample: Comorbidity and associated suicide-related symptoms. *Psychological Medicine*, *30*, 797–804. doi:10.1017/S0033291799002275

Nepon, J., Belik, S., Bolton, J., & Sareen, J. (2010). The relationship between anxiety disorders and suicide attempts: Findings from the national epidemiologic survey on alcohol and related conditions. *Journal of Depression and Anxiety, 27*(9), 791–798. doi:10.1002/da.20674

Ninan, P. T. (2001). Dissolving the burden of generalized anxiety disorder. *The Journal of Clinical Psychiatry, 62*, 5–10.

Nock, M. K., & Kessler, R. C. (2006). Prevalence of and risk factors for suicide attempts versus suicide gestures: Analysis of the national comorbidity survey. *Journal of Abnormal Psychology, 115*(3), 616–623. doi:10.1037/0021-843X.115.3.616

Norton, P. J., Temple, S. R., & Pettit, J. W. (2008). Suicidal ideation and anxiety disorders: Elevator risk or artifact of comorbid depression? *Journal of Behavior Therapy and Experimental Psychiatry, 29*(4), 515–525. doi:10.1016/j.jbtep.2007.10.010

Noyes, R. (1991). Suicide and panic disorder: A review. *Journal of Affective Disorders, 22* (1–2), 1–11. doi:10.1016/0165-0327(91)90077-6

Nutt, D., Argyropoulos, S., Hood, S., & Potokar, J. (2006). Generalized anxiety disorder: A comorbid disease. *European Neuropsychopharmacology, 16*, 109–118. doi:10.1016/j.euroneuro.2006.04.003

O'Connor, R. C., & Nock, M. K. (2014). The psychology if suicidal behavior. *The Lancet Psychiatry, 1*(1), 73–85. doi:10.1016/S2215-0366(14)70225-1

Ohring, R., Apter, A., Ratzoni, G., Weizman, R., Tyano, S., & Plutchik, R. (1996). State and trait anxiety in adolescent suicide attempters. *Child Adolescent Psychiatry, 35*(2), 154–157.

Olatunji, B. O., Cisler, J. M., & Tolin, D. F. (2007). Quality of life in the anxiety disorders: A meta-analytic review. *Clinical Psychological Review, 27*(5), 572–581. doi:10.1016/j.cpr.2007.01.015

Overbeek, T., Rikken, J., Schruers, K., & Griez, E. (1998). Suicidal ideation in panic disorder patients. *Journal of Nervous Mental Disorders, 186*, 577–580. doi:10.1097/00005053-199809000-00010

Peles, E., Schrieber, S., & Adleson, M. (2009). Association of OCD with a history of traumatic events among patients in methadone maintenance treatment. *CNS Spectrums, 14*(10), 547–554. doi:10.1017/S1092852900024032

Pettit, J. W., Buitron, V., & Green, K. L. (2018). Assessment and management of suicide risk in children and adolescents. *Cognitive Behavioral Practice, 25*(4), 460–472.

Philips, K. A., Pinto, A., Menard, W., Eisen, J. L., Mancebo, M., & Rasmussen, S. A. (2007). The clinical impact of bipolar and unipolar affective comorbidity on obsessive-compulsive disorder. *Journal of Affective Disorders, 46*, 15–23.

Pine, D. S., Cohen, P., & Gurley, D. (1998). The risk for early-adulthood anxiety and depressive disorders in adolescents with anxiety and depressive disorders. *Archives of General Psychiatry, 55*, 56. doi:10.1001/archpsyc.55.1.56

Portzky, G., Audenaert, K., & van Heeringen, K. (2009). Psychosocial and psychiatric factors associated with adolescent suicide: A case-control psychological autopsy study. *Journal of Adolescence, 32*(4), 849–862. doi:10.1016/j.adolescence.2008.10.007

Rice, T., & Sher, L. (2015). Educating health care trainees and professionals about suicide prevention in depressed adolescents. *International Journal of Adolescent Medicine and Health (3)*, 221–229.

Ritter, V., Ertel, C., Beil, K., Steffens, M. C., & Stangier, U. (2013). In the presence of social threat: Implicit and explicit self-esteem in social anxiety disorder. *Cognitive Therapy and Research, 37*(6), 110–1109. doi:10.1007/s10608-013-9553-0

Rudd, M. D., Dahmn, P. F., & Rajab, M. H. (1993). Diagnostic comorbidity in persons with suicidal ideation and behavior. *American Journal of Psychiatry, 150*(6), 928–934. doi:10.1176/ajp.150.6.928

Rutter, P. A., & Behrendt, A. E. (2004). Adolescent suicide risk: Four psychosocial factors. *Adolescence*, *39*, 295–302.

Sareen, J. (2011). Anxiety disorders and risk for suicide: Why such controversy? *Depression and Anxiety*, *25*, 941–945. doi:10.1002/da.20906

Sareen, J., Cox, B. J., Afifi, T. O., De Graaf, R., Asmundson, G. J. G., Ten Have, M., & Stein, M. B. (2005). Anxiety disorders and risk for suicidal ideation and suicide attempts: A population-based longitudinal study of adults. *Archives of General Psychiatry*, *62*, 1249–1257. doi:10.1001/archpsyc.62.11.1249

Sareen, J., Houlahan, T., Cox, B. J., & Asmundson, G. J. G. (2005). Anxiety disorders associated with suicidal ideation and suicide attempts in the national comorbidity survey. *Journal of Nervous and Mental Disease*, *193*(7), 450–454. doi:10.1097/01.nmd.0000168263.89652.6b

Schmidt, N. B., Wollaway-Bickel, K., & Bates, M. (2005). Evaluating panic-specific factors in the relationship between suicide and panic disorder. *Behaviour Research and Therapy*, *39*(6), 635–649.

Schnika, K. C., Van Dulmen, M. H. M., Bossarte, R., & Swahn, M. (2012). Association between loneliness and suicidality during middle childhood and adolescence: Longitudinal effects of the role of demographic characteristics. *The Journal of Psychology: Interdisciplinary and Applied*, *146*, 105–118. doi:10.1080/00223980.2011.584084

Sheftall, A. H., Asti, L., Horowitz, L. M., Felts, A., Fontanella, C. A., Campo, J. V., & Bridge, J. A. (2016). Suicide in elementary school-aged children in early adolescents. *American Academy of Pediatrics*, *138*.

Sherbourne, C. D., & Wells, K. B. (1997). Course of depression in patients with comorbid anxiety disorders. *Journal of Affective Disorders*, *43*, 245–250. doi:10.1016/S0165-0327(97)01442-0

Shneidman, E. S. (1993). Commentary: Suicide as psychache. *Journal of Nervous and Mental Disease*, *181*(3), 145–147. doi:10.1097/00005053-199303000-00001

Shores, M. M., Glubin, T., Cowley, D. S., Dager, S. R., Roy-Byrne, P. P., & Dunner, D. L. (1992). The relationship between anxiety and depression: A clinical comparison of generalized anxiety disorder, dysthymic disorder, panic disorder, and major depressive disorder. *Comprehensive Psychiatry*, *33*(4), 237–244. doi:10.1016/0010-440X(92)90047-T

Silverman, M. M., Berman, A. L., Sanddal, N. D., O'Carroll, P. W., & Joiner, T. E. (2007). Rebuilding the tower of babel: A revised nomenclature for the study of suicide and suicidal behaviors part 1: Background, rationale, and methodology. *Suicide and Life-Threatening Behavior*, *37*(3), 248–263. doi:10.1521/suli.2007.37.6.671

Storr, C. L., Ialongo, N. S., Anthony, J. C., & Breslau, N. (2007). Childhood antecedents of exposure to traumatic events and posttraumatic stress disorder. *American Journal of Psychiatry*, *164*(1), 119–125. doi:10.1176/ajp.2007.164.5.712

Strauss, J., Birmaher, B., Bridge, J., Axelson, D., Chiappetta, L., Brent, D., & Ryan, N. (2000). Anxiety disorders in suicidal youth. *Canadian Journal of Psychiatry*, *45*, 739–745. doi:10.1177/070674370004500807

Swahn, M. H., & Bossart, R. M. (2007). Gender, early alcohol use, and suicide ideation and attempts: Findings from the 2005 youth risk behavior survey. *Journal of Adolescent Health*, *41*(2), 175–181. doi:10.1016/j.jadohealth.2007.05.016

Teo, A. R., Lerrigo, R., & Rogers, M. A. M. (2013). The role of social isolation in social anxiety disorder: A systematic review and meta-analysis. *Journal of Anxiety Disorders*, *27*(4), 353–364. doi:10.1016/j.janxdis.2013.03.010

Thibodeau, M. A., Welch, P. G., Sareen, J., & Asmundson, G. J. G. (2013). Anxiety disorders are independently associated with suicide ideation and attempts: Propensity score matching in two epidemiological samples. *Journal of Depression and Anxiety*, *30*(10), 947–954. doi:10.1002/da.22203

Torres, A. R., de Abreu Ramos-Cerqueira, A. T., Torresan, R. C., de Souza Domingues, M., Hercos, A. C., & Guimaraes, A. B. (2007). Prevalence and associated factors for suicidal ideation and behaviors in obsessive-compulsive disorder. *CNS Spectrums*, *12*(10), 771–778. doi:10.1017/S1092852900015467

Torres, A. R., Shavitt, R. G., Torresan, R. C., Ferrao, Y. A., Mighel, E. C., & Fontenelle, L. F. (2013). Clinical features of pure obsessive-compulsive disorder. *Comprehensive Psychiatry*, *54*(7), 1042–1052. doi:10.1016/j.comppsych.2013.04.013

Vaele, D., & Roberts, A. (2014). Obsessive-compulsive disorder. *BMJ*, *348*, g2183. doi:10.1136/bmj.g2183

Valentiner, D. P., Gutierrez, P. M., & Blacker, D. (2002). Anxiety measures and their relationship to adolescent suicidal ideation and behavior. *Anxiety Disorders*, *16*, 11–32. doi:10.1016/S0887-6185(01)00086-X

Van Orden, K. A., Cukrowicz, K. C., Witte, T. K., & Joiner, T. E., Jr. (2012). Thwarted belongingness and perceived burdensomeness: Construct validity and psychometric properties of the interpersonal needs questionnaire. *Psychological Assessment*, *24*(1), 197–215. doi:10.1037/a0025358

Wei, T., Kutcher, S., & LeBlanc, J. C. (2015). Hot idea or hotair: A systematic review of evidence for two widely marketed youth suicide prevention programs and recommendations for implementation. *Journal of The Canadian Academy of Child and Adolescent Psychiatry*, *24*, 1.

Weissman, M. M., Klerman, G. L., Markoqitz, J. S., & Ouellette, R. (1989). Suicidal ideation and suicide attempts in panic disorder and attacks. *New England Journal of Medicine*, *321* (1), 1209–1214. doi:10.1056/NEJM198911023211801

Wilcox, H. C., Storr, C. L., & Breslau, N. (2009). Post-traumatic stress disorder and suicide attempts in a community sample of urban young American adults. *Archives of General Psychiatry*, *66*(3), 305–311. doi:10.1001/archgenpsychiatry.2008.557

Zimmerman, M., & Chelminski, I. (2003). Generalized anxiety disorder in patients with major depression: Is DMS-IV's hierarchy correct? *American Journal of Psychiatry*, *160*, 504–512. doi:10.1176/appi.ajp.160.3.504

Sleep patterns and anxiety in children interact to predict later suicidal ideation

Priel Meir, Candice A. Alfano, Simon Lau, Ryan M. Hill, and Cara A. Palmer

ABSTRACT

Elevated levels of childhood anxiety pose risk for suicide; however, factors that accentuate this risk are unknown. Seventy-one children participated in a longitudinal study investigating anxiety and sleep in childhood (between 7–11 years) and later suicidal ideation (SI; $M = 3.3$ years later). Sleep was assessed via subjective reports and objective measures (actigraphy and polysomnography). Children with greater anxiety symptoms were at greater risk for later SI when sleep disturbances were present in childhood. Results suggest that sleep disruption may amplify SI risk in anxious children.

Introduction

Suicide is the second leading cause of death among young people across the world (World Health Organization, 2018) and is a serious public health concern. Suicidal ideation (SI) and suicide attempts are also frequent during adolescence, with nearly 30% of adolescents reporting a lifetime history of SI and nearly 10% reporting a lifetime history of suicide attempts (Evans, Hawton, Rodham, & Deeks, 2005). Importantly, many children and teens do not seek or receive help for SI or suicidal behaviors (Gould et al., 2009; Pisani et al., 2012; Schmeelk-Cone, Pisani, Petrova, & Wyman, 2012). Identifying malleable risk factors that can be identified before the onset of suicidal behaviors or ideation by health officials and professionals is critical for early prevention. Anxiety is one risk factor that has been cross-sectionally associated with suicidal behaviors in childhood and adolescence (Hill, Castellanos, & Pettit, 2011). However, studies examining longitudinal associations between anxiety and SI are limited, as are studies examining synergistic risk factors that may buffer or heighten risk for SI in anxious children. The current study examines how sleep disturbances, a common symptom in anxious children that is independently associated with risk for suicide, moderates associations between pre-pubertal anxiety symptoms and later experiences of SI.

Anxiety and suicide

Results from several investigations suggest that anxious individuals are at heightened risk for SI. In a population-based sample of adult primary care patients with anxiety (i.e., met DSM-IV criteria for at least one anxiety disorder and expressed moderate anxiety symptoms), 26% expressed passive SI, 16% held thoughts of suicide within the month of assessment, and 18% expressed a previous history of non-lethal suicide attempt (Bomyea et al., 2013). In adults, Sareen et al. (2005) found that of their participants who endorsed suicidal attempt and suicidal ideation, 55% and 37% of those participants respectively had at least 1 anxiety disorder (i.e., met DSM-III-R criteria). In adolescence, research has demonstrated that subthreshold-anxious and clinically-anxious adolescents are 1.79 and 2.76 times more likely to endorse SI respectively than their non-anxious peers (Balazs et al., 2013). In addition to these compelling cross-sectional associations, a recent meta-analytic study concluded that anxiety was a significant longitudinal predictor of SI and attempts but not suicide completion (Bentley et al., 2016). In an in-patient psychiatric sample of adolescents, Goldston et al. (1999) identified trait anxiety symptoms as associated with suicide attempts 5 years later. Another longitudinal study in adolescents observed that teens with current SI were significantly more likely to have previously endorsed anxiety symptoms in childhood than their non-suicidal peers (Reinherz et al., 1995). Further, in adolescents aged 7–14 years treated with cognitive-behavioral therapy for a primary anxiety disorder who were followed-up 7–19 years later, 27.3% endorsed either current or lifetime SI, with treatment non-responders being significantly more likely to have endorsed SI at follow-up (Wolk, Kendall, & Beidas, 2015). Importantly, studies have shown that this relationship between anxiety and later suicide risk exists over and above other comorbidities (e.g., depression; Boden, Fergusson, & Horwood, 2007).

Conversely, other studies have not found the presence of an anxiety disorder prior to puberty to pose increased suicide risk (Weissman et al., 1999; Wolk & Weissman, 1996). In addition, despite evidence for longitudinal relations between anxiety and suicide attempts and ideation, effect sizes are generally small (Bentley et al., 2016). Other limitations of this body of research include the fact that few studies have examined anxiety symptoms prior to the onset of puberty, and many studies have examined anxiety diagnoses or symptoms in isolation (i.e., without accounting for comorbid symptoms). As anxiety is highly comorbid with a range of other conditions and symptoms, it is unknown whether and how anxiety might interact with other established risk factors in the development of later SI. As a result, our current understanding of which anxious children are most at-risk for later SI is inadequate. One established risk factor that likely impacts later SI and disproportionately impacts anxious children is sleep disturbances. Investigation into how particular sleep patterns early in life may accentuate or buffer suicide risk in anxious children and adolescents is needed.

Anxiety and sleep disturbances in childhood and adolescence

Sleep patterns are an important risk factor to consider when examining psychiatric outcomes in anxious children for several reasons. First, a majority of children with clinical levels of anxiety experience subjective sleep complaints (McMakin & Alfano, 2015), including difficulties at bedtime (e.g., problems initiating sleep, bedtime resistance), maintaining sleep throughout the night, and poor sleep quality (e.g., feeling rested upon waking in the morning). Sleep onset is also mildly prolonged based on assessments using actigraphy (Alfano, 2018). Second, the presence of sleep disturbances is associated with more severe forms of anxiety and greater impairments in functioning (Alfano, Ginsburg, & Kingery, 2007; Chase & Pincus, 2011). Additionally, certain aspects of sleep architecture have been shown to correlate with symptom profiles among anxious children. Palmer and Alfano (2017a) found a greater percentage of rapid eye movement (REM) sleep to correspond with greater depressive symptoms whereas lower percentages of non-REM (NREM) stage 3 sleep (i.e., slow wave sleep) was associated with greater negative affect for anxious children but not healthy controls. These collective findings suggest both subjective and objective sleep characteristics to hold meaning for the emotional experiences of anxious children. Lastly, better understanding of potentially synergistic relationships between anxiety and sleep across the transition from childhood to adolescence, a period when both sleep and emotional systems are changing, has been highlighted as a critical area for research inquiry (Alfano, 2018; McMakin & Alfano, 2015).

Sleep and suicide

Several longitudinal studies and meta-analyses provide evidence for subjective sleep disturbances (e.g., insomnia, nightmares) as an independent risk-factor for suicidality in adults despite different methodologies, sample demographics, and when controlling for the effects of depression and other comorbid symptoms (Bernert, Kim, Iwata, & Perlis, 2015; Fujino, Mizoue, Tokui, & Yoshimura, 2005; Nadorff, Anestis, Nazem, Harris, & Winer, 2014; Pigeon, Pinquart, & Conner, 2012; Tanskanen et al., 2001; Turvey et al., 2002). In children and adolescents, previous studies suggest that those who endorsed SI or suicidal attempt were more likely to have sleep problems compared to those who did not endorse SI or attempt (Franic, Kralj, Marcinko, Knez, & Kardum, 2014; Gex, Narring, Ferron, & Michaud, 1998; Liu, 2004; Vignau et al., 1997). However, published literature examining longitudinal relationships between sleep disturbances and suicidality in children and adolescents is unfortunately limited (Liu & Buysse, 2006). One study using a large ($N = 6{,}504$) sample of adolescents found that sleep difficulties (i.e., difficulty falling asleep, nocturnal wakefulness) predicted both suicidal attempts and ideation one and five years later (Wong & Brower, 2012). One other longitudinal study using an adolescent sample has similarly found significant relationships between sleep disturbances and both SI and non-lethal suicide attempt several years later, even when controlling for age, gender, depressive symptoms, aggressive behavior, and substance abuse (Wong, Brower, & Zucker, 2011).

Importantly, the aforementioned longitudinal studies relied on subjective reports of sleep without additionally incorporating objective measures (i.e., actigraphy, polysomnography). Research using polysomnography among adults has shown marked differences in the sleep patterns of those endorsing suicidality and those who do not, with the most reliable differences emerging for patterns of REM sleep. For example, one study found greater REM sleep and phasic REM activity (along with a longer sleep onset latency) among depressed adults endorsing suicidality as compared to depressed adults without a history of suicide (Sabo, Reynolds III, Kupfer, & Berman, 1990). Similar findings have been reported among adults with schizophrenia (Lewis et al., 1996) and untreated depression (Agargun & Cartwright, 2003). Additional research using polysomnography found current SI in adult patients with either major depressive disorder or bipolar disorder was significantly associated with less NREM sleep and higher nocturnal wakefulness when controlling for depressive symptoms (Bernert et al., 2017).

Within adolescent populations, research using objective sleep data is more limited and somewhat mixed. Increased slow wave sleep and the interaction between slow wave and altered REM sleep during adolescence has been found to predict suicidality 10–15 years later (Goetz, Wolk, Coplan, Ryan, & Weissman, 2001). Comparatively, Dahl et al. (1990) examined polysomnography sleep measures in adolescents with major depressive disorder with and without SI. The adolescents with SI had significantly longer sleep onset latencies than their non-suicidal peers, but differences in REM latency, REM density, or REM time were not found (Dahl et al., 1990). Other research comparing polysomnography sleep measures in adolescents with major depressive disorder did not find differences between those who endorsed SI and those who did not (Rao et al., 1996).

The current study

In sum, a growing number of studies provide evidence that both anxiety and aspects of sleep are prospectively associated with risk for SI. However, interactions between childhood anxiety and sleep in predicting suicidal ideation have yet to be examined, and studies examining both subjective and objective sleep patterns and longitudinal predictors of SI in childhood are limited. Investigation of early sleep patterns that might modify SI risk for anxious children and adolescents could help identify those most vulnerable. This longitudinal study aimed to address these gaps using both subjective reports and objective measures of sleep in a sample of pre-pubertal children with a range of anxiety symptoms. These participants underwent a second assessment approximately 3 to 4 years later. It was hypothesized that greater anxiety symptoms at Time 1 would predict elevated risk for SI at Time 2, and that the presence of subjective sleep disturbances in childhood would amplify SI risk. Also, based on findings in adults showing greater nighttime wakings (Wong & Brower, 2012), increased sleep onset latency (Dahl et al., 1990; Wong & Brower, 2012), and increased REM sleep (Agargun & Cartwright, 2003; Lewis et al., 1996) to forecast SI risk, we hypothesized the same relationships in our sample of children.

Methods

Participants included 71 children who completed a comprehensive sleep and psychiatric assessment between the ages of 7–11 years, and a follow-up assessment approximately 3–4 years later (M = 3.34, SD = 1.63, range 1–7). All children were pre-pubertal at Time 1 as determined by the Pubertal Development Scale (PDS; Carskadon & Acebo, 1993). Participant demographic characteristics are displayed in Table 1.

Inclusion/exclusion criteria

Participants were recruited at Time 1 to capture a range of both clinical and subclinical anxiety symptoms. To be eligible to participate at Time 1, children were required to live with a primary caretaker, be fluent in English (and have a caretaker who was fluent in English), and could not be taking medications or over the counter supplements known to impact anxiety or sleep (e.g., melatonin, selective serotonin reuptake inhibitors). Participants also could not have any chronic medical conditions that might impact their sleep (e.g., atopic dermatitis) or any diagnosed or suspected organic sleep disorders (e.g., sleep apnea, restless leg syndrome). Because the purpose of the study was to investigate relationships between anxiety and sleep specifically, children were also excluded if they had any lifetime or current history of depressive disorders. In addition, children with psychotic, pervasive developmental, or bipolar disorders, and/or any lifetime presence of suicidal behaviors or ideation were ineligible at Time 1. Parents reported on all of these exclusionary criteria during a phone screening assessment prior to their participation. Participants also underwent polysomnography to further assess for the presence of any sleep disorders, and completed testing to ensure that they did not have an IQ below 80 (which was confirmed using the Wechsler

Table 1. Demographic characteristics and between-group comparisons for participants reporting (n = 16) and not reporting (n = 55) SI.

	SI	No SI	Entire Sample		
	M (SD)/n (%)	M (SD)/n (%)	M (SD)/n (%)	t(df) or X^2(df)	p
Age (Time 1)	9.5 (.89)	8.8 (1.49)	8.99 (1.40)	−2.21 (41.41)	.03
Age (Time 2)	12.75 (1.73)	12.18 (2.17)	12.31 (2.08)	−.96 (69)	.34
Sex				5.8 (1)	.02
Male	3 (18.75%)	29 (52.73%)	32 (45.07%)		
Female	13 (81.25%)	26 (47.27%)	39 (54.93%)		
Race				5.1 (4)	.28
White	12 (75%)	34 (61.81%)	46 (64.78%)		
Black/African-American	1 (6.25%)	12 (21.82%)	13 (18.30%)		
Asian	0 (0%)	4 (7.27%)	4 (5.63%)		
Biracial/Other	3 (18.75%)	5 (9.09%)	8 (11.27%)		
Ethnicity				.01 (1)	.93
Hispanic/Latino	6 (37.50%)	20 (36.36%)	26 (36.62%)		
Not Hispanic/Latino	10 (62.50%)	35 (49.30%)	45 (63.80%)		
Diagnoses (Time 1)				6.9 (1)	.01
No Diagnosis	11 (68.75%)	48 (87.27%)	59 (82.10%)		
Social Anxiety	1 (6.25%)	3 (5.45%)	4 (5.63%)		
Specific Phobia	1 (6.25%)	2 (3.64%)	3 (4.23%)		
GAD	4 (25%)	6 (10.91%)	10 (14.08%)		
MDD	0 (0%)	0 (0%)	0 (0%)		
ADHD	0 (0%)	0 (0%)	0 (0%)		
Other	1 (6.25%)	1 (1.82%)	1 (1.41%)		
Diagnoses (Time 2)				4.4 (1)	.04
No Diagnosis	5 (31.25%)	50 (90.9%)	55 (77.46%)		
Social Anxiety	3 (18.75%)	0 (0%)	3 (4.23%)		
Specific Phobia	1 (6.25%)	2 (3.64%)	3 (4.23%)		
GAD	5 (31.25%)	3 (5.45%)	8 (11.27%)		
MDD	3 (18.75%)	0 (0%)	3 (4.23%)		
ADHD	0 (0%)	1 (1.82%)	1 (1.41%)		
Other	1 (6.25%)	2 (3.64%)	3 (4.23%)		
Missing*	1 (6.25%)	0 (0%)	1 (1.41%)		

Notes. SI = suicidal ideation, GAD = generalized anxiety disorder, MDD = major depressive disorder, ADHD = attention-deficit/hyper activity disorder. Many participants met criteria for multiple disorders. Chi-square results for psychiatric diagnoses between the SI group and no SI group compare those who met criteria for any psychiatric disorder compared to those who did not meet criteria for any disorder. *One participant is missing a final diagnosis at Time 2 due to reports of severe ideation during the diagnostic interview, and as a result the assessment was ended early.

Abbreviated Scale of Intelligence; Wechsler, 1999). Diagnostic status and psychiatric history was further assessed using the Anxiety Disorders Interview Schedule for the DSM-IV for Children and Parents (Silverman & Albano, 1996).

Procedure

All study procedures at Time 1 were approved by the Institutional Review Board at the University of Houston. Study procedures for the assessment at Time 2 were approved as a separate follow-up study by the Institutional Review Board. At Time 2, participants were recruited from a larger sample of

96 children who completed a Time 1 assessment as part of one of two studies with nearly identical assessment procedures. One study targeted children with anxiety disorders or healthy children (n = 25) and the other study targeted children with subclinical levels of anxiety (n = 46). All families at Time 1 were recruited using flyers, postcard mailings using public school databases, and through public/community events.

At Time 1, all children and one parent were consented/assented and then completed an initial assessment that included parent-reported questionnaires about the child's sleep and psychiatric symptoms, a diagnostic interview to determine any clinical diagnoses, and abbreviated IQ testing. All children then completed 6–7 days of actigraphy sleep monitoring and one night of at-home polysomnography sleep monitoring. At Time 2, families from Time 1 were contacted and asked if they would like to participate in a separate follow-up study to assess their child's current level of functioning. Interested participants were re-consented/assented and completed one in-person assessment. During this assessment, participants completed both parent and child-reported questionnaires, along with the same diagnostic interview as Time 1. A Ph.D.-level psychologist or a trained doctoral-level graduate student conducted all assessments at both time points.

Assessments

Suicidal ideation (SI)

No children reported SI or self-harm behaviors at Time 1. This was verified during the diagnostic interview, and also by parent-report on the Child Behavior Checklist (CBCL; Achenbach & Rescorla, 2001). At Time 2, participants were dichotomized based on whether they reported any occurrence of SI. This presence of current or previous SI was assessed via either self-report from participants on the Children's Depression Inventory (CDI; Kovacs, 1992) which were then fol-lowed-up by a clinician, or were reported during the diagnostic interview. During the semi-structured diagnostic interview, participants were provided with an initial prompt to assess their experience of depressive symptoms. If participants indicated the presence of depression, they were given a series of follow-up yes or no questions regarding specific symptoms they had experienced, including the experience of suicidal thoughts over the last two weeks. All participants also completed the full 27-item CDI as part of the general study procedures, including one item assessing suicidal ideation. This item on the CDI provides participants with an option to choose one of the following statements describing their feelings and thoughts over the last two weeks: a) *I do not think about killing myself,* b) *I think about killing myself, but I would not do it,* and c) *I want to kill myself.* Children were also provided the option to decline to answer this question. For all participants selecting options b, c, or who declined to answer, further SI assess-ment was conducted through a clinician-administered risk assessment. Any reports of SI (by the parent or participant) during follow-up questions or the diagnostic interview were immediately reviewed with a licensed clinical psychologist to determine risk and next steps. Participants with confirmed suicidal ideation based on the diagnostic interview, the CDI item, and/or these follow-up questions were coded as 1 (*endorsed SI*) and participants without suicidal ideation were coded as 0 (*did not endorse SI*).

Sleep patterns

Subjective reports. Parents reported on their child's sleep patterns at Time 1 using the Children's Sleep Habits Questionnaire (CSHQ; Owens, Spirito, & McGuinn, 2000). The CSHQ includes 33 items that assess a range of various sleep problems. Parents were asked to report how often certain sleep difficulties occurred in a recent typical week of their child's sleep from 1 (*rarely; 0–1 times a week*), 2 (*sometimes; 2–4 times a week*), or 3 (*usually; 5–7 times a week*). The CSHQ includes subscales that assess the following sleep problems: *bedtime resistance* (α = .61, 6 items; e.g., "Child needs parent in the room to fall asleep"), *sleep onset delay* (assessed with one reversed scored item, "Child falls asleep within 20 minutes after going to bed"), *sleep anxiety* (α = .74, 4 items; e.g., "Child has trouble sleeping away from home"), *sleep duration* (α = .74, 3 items; e.g., "Child sleeps too little"), *daytime sleepiness* (α = .82, 8 items; e.g., "Child takes a long time to become alert in the morning"), *sleep disordered breathing* (α = .51, 3 items; e.g., "Child snores loudly"), *night awakenings* (α = .31, 3 items; e.g., "Child awakes more than once during the night"), and *parasomnias* (α = .13, 7 items; e.g., "Child awakens alarmed by a frightening dream"). Reliability analyses indicated that removing one item from the night awakening subscale ("Child moves to someone else's bed during the night") resulted in an increase in Cronbach's alpha from .31 to .61. As a result, the final scores from this subscale included the remaining 2 items only. Due to the exclusionary criteria of the current sample (i.e., no organically based sleep disorders), along with the low internal consistencies, we did not include the parasomnias or sleep disordered breathing subscales. We also calculated a *total sleep disturbance* score (α = .79).

Actigraphy. Actigraphy-based sleep patterns were assessed in childhood using a wrist-based accelerometer (Micro Motionlogger Actigraph Sleep Watches; Ambulatory Monitoring Inc., Ardsley, NY). Participants wore the watch for 6–7 days, and pushed an event button each evening when they got into bed each night, and again in the morning when they got out of bed. Participants were also asked to complete a sleep diary each morning and evening, which is a necessary validation check for actigraphy to confirm sleep-wake times and identify any artifacts or irregularities in the data (Meltzer, Montgomery-Downs, Insana, & Walsh, 2012). Data was visually inspected to omit any epochs where the watch was not worn. Consistent with other studies using actigraphy in pediatric populations, data was scored using the zero-crossing mode and the Sadeh algorithm in one minute epochs (Meltzer et al., 2012; Sadeh, Sharkey, & Carskadon, 1994). The variables derived from the actigraphy estimates include total sleep time (TST, or average minutes of sleep duration), sleep onset latency (SOL, or the number of minutes taken to fall asleep), and wake after sleep onset (WASO, or the number of minutes spent awake at night between sleep onset and sleep offset time). Based on recommendations for using actigraphy in pediatric research, only participants with a minimum of 5 nights of valid data were included in the present analyses (Acebo et al., 1999).

Polysomnography. Children completed one night of unattended, at-home polysomnography monitoring, which included 6 channels of EEG (frontal, central, and occipital regions), along with EOG, facial EMG, electrocardiogram, respiratory inductance plethysmography, pulse oximetry, and tibial EMG. Some participants (n = 25) were prepared for the polysomnography recording at a pediatric sleep center using NicoletOne ambulatory equipment (Natus, Inc.) and some participants (n = 46) were prepared for the recording at their home using RemLogic Embletta equipment (Natus, Inc.). All participants slept at home (based on prescribed bed and wake times) and simultaneously wore actigraph watches. Some participants were missing polysomnography data due to data recording errors, or when actigraphy data indicated that polysomnography did not capture the entire sleep period (i.e., either fell asleep prior to the start of the recording, or slept in after the recording was set to end). These participants (n = 21) were not included in analyses using polysomnography variables. All recordings were reviewed and scored by registered sleep technicians with pediatric experience and reviewed by a certified sleep medicine specialist. Recordings were scored in 30-second epochs using the criteria set forth by the American Academy of Sleep Medicine scoring rules (Iber, Ancoli-Israel, Chesson, & Quan, 2007). For the current study, the polysomnography derived variables included the percentage of total sleep time that was spent in N3 sleep (N3%) and percentage of total sleep time that was spent in REM sleep (REM%).

Psychopathology symptoms
Clinical interview. At both Time 1 and Time 2, participants completed the Anxiety Disorders Interview Schedule for DSM-IV for Children and Parents (ADIS-C/P; Silverman & Albano, 1996), which has excellent psychometric properties (Lyneham, Abbott, & Rapee, 2007; Silverman, Saavedra, & Pina, 2001). Separate interviews were conducted with a caregiver and the child by a Ph.D.-level psychologist or a trained doctoral level graduate student according to standardized procedures. All cases were reviewed with

a licensed clinical psychologist prior to assigning any diagnoses. A summary of the diagnoses at Time 1 and Time 2 are provide in Table 1.

Anxiety symptoms. Child anxiety symptoms were assessed at Time 1 via parent-report on the Child Behavior Checklist (CBCL; Achenbach & Rescorla, 2001). Specifically, parents reported on how much a series of statements described their child now or in the last 6 months from 0 (*not true of their child*) to 2 (*very true or often true of their child*). For the current study, we used the DSM-oriented anxiety subscale. However, this subscale includes one item about sleep which was removed for the purposes of the current study. The remaining 8 items were averaged to create a total anxiety symptoms subscale (α = .81).

Depressive symptoms. Child depressive symptoms at Time 1 were assessed using parent-reported scores on the DSM-oriented depressive symptoms subscale of the CBCL (Achenbach & Rescorla, 2001). Similar to the anxiety subscale, parents responded to statements based on how well they described their child now or in the last 6 months from 0 (*not true of their child*) to 2 (*very true or often true of their child*). For the current study, we removed four items from this subscale that pertained to sleep, and 2 items that pertained to self-harm and SI. The remaining 7 items were averaged to create a total depressive symptoms subscale (α = .41).

Analysis plan

First, a series of chi-squares and t-tests were conducted to determine any potential significant differences between participants reporting and not reporting SI at Time 2. We also examined bivariate associations among other variables of interest and demographic characteristics. Finally, based on the dichotomous nature of our SI outcome, a series of logistic regression models predicting the presence of SI were conducted. All analyses included sleep patterns at Time 1 (either subjective, actigraphy-measured TST, SOL, or WASO, or polysomnography-measured N3% or REM%), anxiety symptoms (based on the CBCL) at Time 1, and the interaction between sleep and anxiety symptoms. These analyses were conducted using the PROCESS 3.1 macro plugin for SPSS (Hayes, 2013). Due to the small number of cases with SI, and the lack of prospective data on sleep and suicide in anxious youth, we set the PROCESS criteria to probe the simple slopes for all interactions with a *p* value of less than .20 to examine exploratory relationships and minimize the possibility of Type II error. All analyses controlled for the time lapse between the two assessments, along with depressive symptoms at Time 1.

Results

Preliminary analyses

A total of 16 participants (22.54%) reported that they experienced SI between Time 1 and Time 2. A summary of the differences between participants who reported SI compared to those who did not endorse SI on all demographic characteristics and variables of interest is reported in Tables 1 and 2. Initial comparisons indicated that participants who did and did not report SI at Time 2 did not differ significantly on any Time 1 sleep variables or Time 1 anxiety or depressive symptoms.

As expected, bivariate analyses indicated that anxiety and depressive symptoms were significantly associated with one another ($r = .52$, $p < .001$). Total subjective sleep disturbances were associated with anxiety ($r = .49$, $p < .001$) and depressive symptoms ($r = .42$, $p < .001$). Anxiety symptoms were associated with several subscales on the CSHQ as well, including greater bedtime resistance ($r = .39$, $p = .001$), sleep onset delay ($r = .45$, $p < .001$), sleep anxiety ($r = .50$, $p < .001$), and greater daytime sleepiness ($r = .34$, $p = .049$). Depressive symptoms were associated with a longer subjective sleep onset delay ($r = .29$, $p = .02$), greater sleep anxiety ($r = .37$, p = .002), daytime sleepiness ($r = .33$, $p = .01$), and total sleep disturbances ($r = .42, p < .001$). There were no significant associations among symptoms and the polysomnography and actigraphy sleep variables.

Table 2. Means, standard deviations, and between-group comparisons between participants reporting (n = 16) and not reporting (n = 55) SI on Time 1 variables.

	SI	No SI	Entire Sample			
	M (SD)	M (SD)	M (SD)	t(df)	p	95% CI
Symptoms						
Anxiety Symptoms	.44(.52)	.22(.25)	.27 (.34)	−2.38(17.12)	.12	−.51, .06
Depressive Symptoms	.15(.14)	.09(.15)	.10 (.15)	−1.45(69)	.15	−.14, .02
Subjective Sleep						
Total Disturbances	44.63(10.07)	41.98(5.88)	42.59 (7.06)	−1.00(18.13)	.33	−8.19, 2.90
Sleep Onset Delay	1.44(.73)	1.31(.54)	1.34(.59)	−.73(68)	.47	−.46, .21
Sleep Duration	3.56(.89)	3.46(.97)	3.49(.94)	−.37(68)	.71	−.64, .44
Night Wakings	2.56(1.21)	2.29(.54)	2.36(.74)	−1.27(68)	.21	−.69, .15
Daytime Sleepiness	12.88(3.56)	12.52 (3.60)	12.60(3.57)	−.35(68)	.73	−2.40, 1.68
Bedtime Resistance	7.88(2.19)	7.44(2.04)	7.54(2.07)	−.73(68)	.47	−1.61, .75
Sleep Anxiety	5.56(2.22)	5.02(1.74)	5.14(1.86)	−1.03(68)	.31	−1.60, .51
Actigraphy						
SOL	20.44(14.87)	21.19 (10.30)	21.01 (11.42)	.22(62)	.83	−6.06, 7.56
TST	508.63(36.28)	505.37(42.54)	506.11 (40.99)	−.28(69)	.78	−26.64, 20.12
WASO	33.27(25.07)	30.58(23.09)	31.20(23.40)	−.40(67)	.69	−16.10, 10.72
PSG						
N3%	23.72 (6.32)	23.06 (7.91)	23.24 (7.47)	−.27(48)	.79	−5.55, 4.23
REM%	18.27 (4.64)	20.01 (6.78)	19.55 (6.29)	.85(48)	.40	−2.34, 5.83

Notes. SI = suicidal ideation, SOL = sleep onset latency (minutes), TST = total sleep time (minutes), WASO = wake after sleep onset (minutes), PSG = polysomnography, N3% = percentage of total sleep comprised of stage 3 sleep, REM% = percentage of total sleep comprised of REM sleep.

Bivariate associations with demographic characteristics indicated that age at Time 1 was associated with less total sleep time measured via actigraphy ($r = -.27$, $p = .02$), and age at Time 2 was associated with shorter subjective sleep duration ($r = .30$, $p = .01$). There were no differences in any variables of interest based on gender, with the exception of SI at Time 2. Girls were significantly more likely to report SI compared to boys, $X^2(1) = 5.78$, $p = .02$ (13 of the 16 SI cases were girls, adjusted residual = 2.4).

Prospective associations between sleep, anxiety, and SI

Logistic regression models were examined with Time 1 anxiety symptoms, Time 1 sleep variables (CSHQ, actigraphy, or polysomnography), and the interaction between Time 1 anxiety and sleep. Models also controlled for the variable time lapse between the two assessments, as well as Time 1 depressive symptoms.

Subjective sleep

For parent-reported total subjective sleep disturbance, the overall model was significant $X^2(5) = 15.81$, $p = .007$. The model as a whole explained between 20.21% (Cox and Snell R squared) and 30.68% (Nagelkerke R squared) of the variance in SI. A significant interaction emerged between Time 1 sleep and anxiety symptoms (Beta = .66, SE = .25, $p = .008$, 95% CI: .17, 1.16), where anxiety predicted a greater likelihood of reporting SI at Time 2 for those with high levels of subjective sleep disturbances ($\text{Effect}_{high} = 6.28$, $\text{SE}_{high} = 2.62$, $p_{high} = .016$, 95% CI_{high}: 1.14, 11.42; $\text{Effect}_{low} = -2.98$, $\text{SE}_{low} = 2.25$, $p_{low} = .19$, 95% CI_{low}: −7.39, 1.44). This interaction is displayed in Figure 1. Follow-up analyses of the simple slopes using the Johnson-Neyman technique indicated that anxiety symptoms were a significant predictor of later SI when sleep disturbances on the CSHQ were at values of 46.47 or above, which is just above the established clinical cut-off score of 41 (Owens et al., 2000).

Follow-up analyses examined the individual subscales of the CSHQ in predicting SI. For parent-reported sleep onset delay, the overall model was significant: $X^2(5) = 14.34$, $p = .01$. The model as a whole explained between 19.06% (Cox and Snell R squared) and 28.12% (Nagelkerke R squared) of the variance in SI. A significant interaction emerged between parent-reported sleep onset delay and anxiety symptoms (Beta = 9.03, SE = 4.03, $p = .025$, 95% CI: 1.12, 16.93), anxiety symptoms predicted a greater likelihood of reporting SI at Time 2 for those with longer sleep onset delay ($\text{Effect}_{long} = 8.05$, $\text{SE}_{long} = 3.60$, $p_{long} = .025$, 95% CI_{long}: .99, 15.11; $\text{Effect}_{short} = -.98$, $\text{SE}_{short} = 1.82$, $p_{short} = .59$, 95% CI_{short}: −4.54, 2.59). This interaction is displayed in Figure 2.

No findings emerged for the bedtime resistance or sleep anxiety subscales of the CSHQ, however several marginal interactions emerged between anxiety and parent-reported sleep duration, night wakings, and daytime sleepiness. For

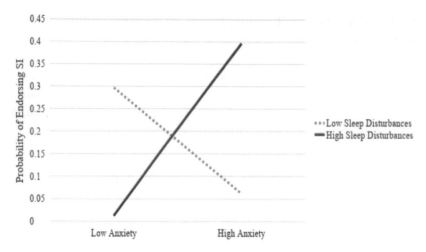

Figure 1. Interaction between anxiety symptoms and subjective sleep disturbances at Time 1 predicting SI at Time 2. The simple slope of high levels of sleep disturbances is significant ($p = .016$).

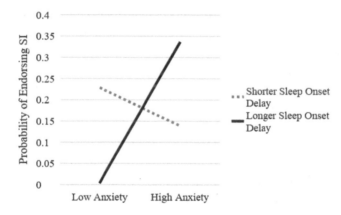

Figure 2. Interaction between anxiety symptoms and subjective sleep onset delay at Time 1 predicting SI at Time 2. The simple slope for a longer sleep onset delay is significant ($p = .025$).

parent-reported sleep duration, the interaction with anxiety symptoms was trending (Beta = 2.34, SE = 1.51, $p = .12$, 95% CI: −.61, 5.30), although the overall model was not significant. The model explained between 11.72% (Cox and Snell R squared) and 17.97% (Nagelkerke R squared) of the variance in SI. Analyses of the simple slopes indicated that for shorter sleep duration but not for longer sleep duration, anxiety was a marginal predictor of later SI (Estimate$_{short}$ = 4.40, SE$_{short}$ = 2.29, p_{short} = .055, 95% CI$_{short}$: −.09, 8.90; Estimate$_{long}$ = .55, SE$_{long}$ = 1.47, p_{long} = .70, 95% CI$_{long}$: −2.33, 3.44). For parent-reported night wakings, the overall model was significant: $X^2(5) = 13.64$, $p = .018$. The model explained between 17.71% (Cox and Snell R squared) and 26.88% (Nagelkerke R squared) of the variance. A marginal interaction between anxiety symptoms and reports of night wakings emerged (Beta = 8.03, SE = 4.74, p = .09, 95% CI: −1.26, 17.33), such that anxiety was marginally associated with a greater likelihood of endorsing SI for those who experienced greater night wakings, but not for those with reports of low levels of night wakings (Estimate$_{high}$ = 8.55, SE$_{high}$ = 4.73, p_{high} = .07, 95% CI$_{high}$: −.72, 17.81; Estimate$_{low}$ = .51, SE$_{low}$ = 1.44, p_{low} = .72, 95% CI$_{low}$: −2.30, 3.32). For parent-reported daytime sleepiness, the overall model was marginal, $X^2(5)$ = 9.62, p = .087, and explained between 12.84% (Cox and Snell R squared) and 19.49% (Nagelkerke R squared) of the variance in SI, and the interaction was trending (Beta = .73, SE = .43, p = .09, 95% CI: −.11, 1.58). Analyses of the simple slopes suggested that anxiety symptoms were associated with later SI for those reporting high levels of daytime sleepiness, but not for those with low levels of daytime sleepiness (Effect$_{high}$ = 5.15, SE$_{high}$ = 2.44, p_{high} = .03, 95% CI$_{high}$: .38, 9.93; Effect$_{low}$ = − .45, SE$_{low}$ = 1.87, p_{low} = .81, 95% CI$_{low}$: −4.12, 3.22). Figures for these marginal interactions can be found in Supplemental File 1.

Actigraphy

For actigraphy-measured SOL, the interaction with anxiety symptoms was trending (Beta = .13, SE = .09, p = .17, 95% CI: −.05, .31), although the overall model was not significant. The model explained between 10.12% (Cox and Snell R squared) and 15.19% (Nagelkerke R squared) of the variance in SI. Analyses of the simple slopes indicated that anxiety was marginally associated with SI when SOL duration was longer (Effect$_{long}$ = 2.88, SE$_{long}$ = 1.71, p_{long} = .09, 95% CI$_{long}$: −.46, 6.22; Effect$_{short}$ = .04, SE$_{short}$ = 1.93, p_{short} = .98, 95% CI$_{short}$: −3.73, 3.82; see figure in Supplemental File 1). No findings emerged for the models examining actigraphy-measured TST or WASO.

Polysomnography

For REM%, the interaction term between REM% and anxiety symptoms was trending (Estimate = .33, SE = .22, p = .13, 95% CI = − .10, .76). However, the overall model was not significant. The model explained between 14.87% (Cox and Snell R squared) and 21.79% (Nagelkerke R squared) of the variance in SI. Analyses of the simple slopes indicated that anxiety symptoms were a significant predictor of later SI for those experiencing high levels of REM sleep but not those with lower levels of REM sleep (Estimate$_{high}$ = 3.90, SE$_{high}$ = 1.90, p_{high} = .04, 95% CI$_{high}$: .17, 7.63; Estimate$_{low}$ = − .42, SE$_{low}$ = 1.95, p_{low} = .82, 95% CI$_{low}$: −4.25, 3.40; see figure in Supplemental File 1). No findings emerged for N3%.

Discussion

Our study fills a critical gap in the literature by examining both objective and subjective sleep characteristics in conjunction with childhood anxiety symptoms in the prediction of SI risk during the transition from childhood to adolescence. Overall findings suggest that certain aspects of childhood sleep, especially parent-reported sleep disturbances, act synergistically with anxiety symptoms to heighten risk for SI years later. These results converge with other longitudinal data revealing anxiety and sleep disturbances to independently forecast later SI, and extend this work by showing anxious children who also experience comorbid sleep problems to be particularly vulnerable. As both anxiety and sleep problems represent malleable risk factors, these findings also highlight potential opportunity for early identification and prevention.

In terms of subjective sleep reports, results indicated childhood anxiety symptoms were associated with later SI only for children who experienced high levels of sleep disturbance. Notably, an anxiety by sleep interaction was prognostic when total sleep disturbance scores on the CSHQ were above the established clinical cut-off, supporting the clinical utility of this measure. Follow-up analyses of the CSHQ subscales further revealed long sleep onset delays, and marginal evidence for short sleep duration, greater nighttime wakings, and/or daytime sleepiness to pose SI risk in the face of elevated anxiety levels. While some of these interactions or simple slopes were only statistically marginal, it is notable that the patterns of findings were consistent across these subscales.

There are a range of mechanisms that could explain why subjective sleep disturbances amplify anxiety-based risk for SI. For example, negative emotional experiences (Palmer & Alfano, 2017b), problems with cognitive control including increased catastrophizing and rumination (Noone et al., 2014; Carney, Edinger, Meyer, Lindman, & Istre, 2006), and impaired social functioning (Beattie, Kyle, Espie, & Biello, 2015), are exacerbated when sleep is disrupted. Importantly, the current sample was pre-pubertal at Time 1, and sleep-anxiety links may be particularly problematic during the transition to adolescence when emotional systems are developing. Indeed, research has suggested that sleep problems during the early adolescent period may be a time when emotional health is most sensitive to the effects of poor sleep (Kelly & El-Sheikh, 2014). Consequently, it is possible that sleep disturbances may result in cascading negative emotional effects that become more severe overtime. It is also possible that sleep disturbances exacerbate anxiety symptoms in children (Alfano et al., 2007), or lead to the emergence of new symptoms overtime (e.g., depressive symptoms).

Another possible mechanism for associations found among anxiety symptoms, subjective sleep disturbances, and SI is articulated in Joiner's interpersonal-psychological theory of suicide (Joiner, 2005). This theory states that desire to die by suicide may result from perceptions of decreased belongingness and isolation. Many anxious children experience difficulties with social and interpersonal functioning (Beidel & Alfano, 2011) and it increasingly clear that poor sleep similarly also corresponds in a range of social impairments including less time spent engaging in social activities (Beattie et al., 2015; Palmer & Alfano,

2017b). As a result, a combination of anxiety and impairing sleep problems may result in poorer social relationships and ultimately feeling less belongingness. However, as belongingness was not assessed in the current study, this is speculative and these connections should be tested in future investigations.

Joiner's (2005) interpersonal-psychological theory of suicide may also be one possible explanation for the discrepancies between some of the sleep findings. Specifically, marginal findings emerged suggesting that parent-reported sleep duration and night wakings moderated the anxiety-SI relationship, whereas similar objectively measured sleep patterns (TST, WASO) did not. According to the interpersonal-psychological theory of suicide, risk of suicide is greater in those who perceive the self as a burden to others. It is possible that parent-reported sleep disturbances more accurately assess the burden of the child's sleep disturbance on the family, as parents may be more aware of these sleep patterns when they result in some type of disturbance in their own sleep (e.g., their child wakes up throughout the night and requires a parent to help them fall back asleep). As a result, parental reports of sleep problems may be a proxy for perceived burdensomeness of these disturbances. Again, while these connections are largely speculative as burdensomeness was not directly assessed, further examination of the association between parental reports and children's perceptions of their sleep problems as a burden on others may be an important direction for future research. Further, a combination of these potential mechanisms may best explain associations between anxiety, sleep, and suicidal ideation. A recent study of adolescents identified serial indirect effects from anxiety to depressive symptoms to perceived burdensomeness, and finally, to suicide ideation (Hill, Del Busto, Buitron, & Pettit, 2018). It is possible that sleep disturbances impact that pathway at multiple points.

It is also important to note that previous studies using the CSHQ have also identified that the subscales do not directly map on to polysomnography or actigraphy-measured variables (Markovich, Gendron, & Corkum, 2015). Discrepancy between subjective and objective sleep findings may therefore be due to the two methodologies measuring different aspects of sleep disturbances. For example, while actigraphy-measured TST and WASO identify the total time asleep or awake (in minutes), the subjective reports may instead be assessing how problematic these aspects of sleep are for overall sleep health which can be biased by individual differences in sensitivity to sleep need and the disruptiveness of night wakings.

The findings from the present study also contribute to research using polysomnography to determine relationships between sleep and SI. Previous studies have reported associations between increased REM sleep duration and risk for SI in adults (Lewis et al., 1996; Sabo et al., 1990), but not in adolescents (Dahl et al., 1990; Rao et al., 1996). Consistent with prior findings in adolescents, REM% in the present pre-pubertal sample did not significantly predict later ideation. However, it is important to note that the interaction between REM% and anxiety symptoms was trending, and follow-up analyses of the simple slopes indicated that the relationship between anxiety symptoms and SI was significant for those experiencing higher levels of REM%. Longitudinal data on objective sleep characteristics and suicide risk is limited, particularly for anxious children and adolescents, and the findings of this study provide preliminary evidence for these processes. However, this marginal finding should be interpreted with caution until replicated using a larger sample.

The present study has a few limitations that should be acknowledged and considered when planning future research. First, the results of this study should be interpreted with caution due to the small sample size, and further replication is needed in understanding the processes underlying sleep disturbances and SI in anxious children. Consistent with prior research (Redfield et al., 2018), the majority of our participants reporting SI were also primarily female, but our small sample size limited power to test differences by gender. Future studies should further investigate how gender interacts with both childhood anxiety and sleep in predicting later risk. Additionally, our measurement of suicidality was not comprehensive. While all reports of SI were confirmed by a trained interviewer and were reviewed with a licensed clinical psychologist, the nature of our suicide assessment necessitated dichotomizing participants based on whether they reported any SI or no SI. Future studies should measure SI using more comprehensive methods to capture variation in SI severity, such as the Beck Scale for Suicide Ideation (Beck & Steer, 1991) which has demonstrated excellent psychometric properties (Batterham et al., 2015). Additionally, children with SI at Time 1 were excluded from study participation, thus the study was unable to examine children with ideation prior to study entry. Future research should assess suicide risk with greater precision to facilitate more accurate examination of time of onset and course of SI with regard to sleep problems.

The polysomnography data acquired included only a single night of assessment. This limits the assessment as the results may have been biased by first night effects (i.e., discomfort due to electrode placement) or sleep patterns that were not typical or normative of the participants. However, it is important to note that the disruptive effects may have been alleviated slightly as participants slept in their own homes (as opposed to a hospital or sleep laboratory) for the night of the assessment. Lastly, while our sample was somewhat diverse, participants in this study were still predominantly Caucasian/White, limiting the external validity with which the findings may be generalized to other populations. It is highly recommended that future studies seek more diverse participants by exploring these processes in different racial or ethnic groups.

Implications for practice

Identification of early risk for suicide is critical, particularly in high-risk samples (i.e., those with elevated anxiety symptoms). Results from the current study suggest that children with higher pre-pubertal anxiety symptoms were most likely to report SI years later, but only when high levels of sleep disturbance were also present. Based on these findings and previous literature, it is suggested that the incorporation of sleep assessments such as the CSHQ may be an important evidence-based tool in assessing risk for SI. Further, behavioral treatments for childhood sleep disturbances (CBT-I) have been shown to be effective for those who are anxious (Gregory & Sadeh, 2016). Thus, identifying and treating sleep disturbances prior to the onset of adolescence may be an effective treatment in reducing the risk of SI in populations at heightened risk for suicidality.

Disclosure statement

No potential conflict of interest was reported by the authors.

Funding

This work was supported by the National Science Foundation under Grant 1813574 (PI: Palmer); National Institutes of Health under Grant K23 MH081188 (PI: Alfano); and National Institutes of Health under Grant R21 MH099351 (PI: Alfano).

References

Acebo, C., Sadeh, A., Seifer, R., Tzischinsky, O., Wolfson, A. R., Hafer, A., & Carskadon, M. A. (1999). Estimating sleep patterns with activity monitoring in children and adolescents: How many nights are necessary for reliable measures? *Sleep*, *22*(1), 95–103. doi:10.1093/sleep/22.1.95

Achenbach, T. M., & Rescorla, L. A. (2001). Reliability, internal consistency, cross-informant agreement, and stability. In *Manual for the ASEBA school-age forms & profiles* (pp. 99–135). Burlington, VT: University of Vermont, Research Center for Children, Youth, & Families.

Agargun, M. Y., & Cartwright, R. (2003). REM sleep, dream variables and suicidality in depressed patients. *Psychiatry Research*, *119*, 33–39. doi:10.1016/S0165-1781(03)00111-2

Alfano, C. A. (2018). (Re)Conceptualizing sleep among children with anxiety disorders. *Where to Next? Clinical Child and Family Psychology Review*, *16*, 3. doi:10.1007/s10567-018-0267-4

Alfano, C. A., Ginsburg, G. S., & Kingery, J. N. (2007). Sleep-related problems among children and adolescents with anxiety disorders. *Journal of the American Academy of Child and Adolescent Psychiatry*, *46*(2), 224–232. doi:10.1097/01.chi.0000242233.06011.8e

Batterhan, C. J., Ftanou, M., Pirkis, J., Brewer, J. L., Mackinnon, A. J., Beautrais, A., Fairweather-Schmidt, A. K., & Christensen, H. (2015). A systematic review and evaluation of measures for suicidal ideation and behaviors in population-based research. *Psychological Assessment, 27*, 501–512.

Beattie, L., Kyle, S. D., Espie, C. A., & Biello, S. M. (2015). Social interactions, emotion and sleep: A systematic review and research agenda. *Sleep Medicine Reviews, 24*, 83–100. doi:10.1016/j.smrv.2014.12.005

Beck, A., & Steer, R. (1991). *Manual for the beck scale for suicide ideation.* San Antonio, TX: Psychological Corporation.

Beidel, D. C., & Alfano, C. A. (2011). *Childhood anxiety disorders: A guide to research and treatment (2nd edition).* New York, NY: Taylor & Francis/Routledge Mental Health.

Bentley, K. H., Franklin, J. C., Ribeiro, J. D., Kleiman, E. M., Fox, K. R., & Nock, M. K. (2016). Anxiety and its disorders as risk factors for suicidal thoughts and behaviors: A meta-analytic review. *Clinical Psychology Review, 43*, 30–46. doi:10.1016/j.cpr.2015.11.008

Bernert, R. A., Kim, J. S., Iwata, N. G., & Perlis, M. L. (2015). Sleep disturbances as an evidence-based suicide risk factor. *Current Psychiatry Reports, 17*(15). doi:10.1007/s11920-015-0552-4

Bernert, R. A., Luckenbaugh, D. A., Duncan, W. C., Iwata, N. G., Ballard, E. D., & Zarate, C. A. (2017). Sleep architecture parameters as a putative biomarker of suicidal ideation in treatment-resistant depression. *Journal of Affective Disorders, 208*, 309–315. doi:10.1016/j.jad.2016.08.050

Boden, J. M., Fergusson, D. M., & Horwood, L. J. (2007). Anxiety disorders and suicidal behaviors in adolescence and young adulthood: Findings from a longitudinal study. *Psychological Medicine, 37*, 431–440. doi:10.1017/S0033291706009147

Bomyea, J., Lang, A. J., Craske, M. G., Chavira, D., Sherbourne, C. D., Rose, R. D., ... Stein, M. B. (2013). Suicidal ideation and risk factors in primary care patients with anxiety disorders. *Psychiatry Research, 209*, 60–65. doi:10.1016/j.psychres.2013.03.017

Carney, C. E., Edinger, J. D., Meyer, B., Lindman, L., & Istre, T. (2006). Symptom-focused rumination and sleep disturbance. *Behavioral Sleep Medicine, 4*(4), 228–241. doi:10.1207/s15402010bsm0404_3

Carskadon, M. A., & Acebo, C. (1993). A self-administered rating scale for pubertal development. *Journal of Adolescent Health, 14*(3), 190–195. doi:10.1016/1054-139X(93)90004-9

Chase, R. M., & Pincus, D. B. (2011). Sleep-related problems in children and adolescents with anxiety disorders. *Behavioral Sleep Medicine, 9*(4), 224–236. doi:10.1080/15402002.2011.606768

Dahl, R. E., Puig-Antich, J., Ryan, N. D., Nelson, B., Dachille, S., Cunningham, S. L., ... Klepper, T. P. (1990). EEG sleep in adolescents with major depression: The role of suicidality and inpatient status. *Journal of Affective Disorders, 19*, 63–75.

Evans, E., Hawton, K., Rodham, K., & Deeks, J. (2005). The prevalence of suicidal phenomena in adolescents: A systematic review of population-based studies. *Suicide and Life-Threatening Behavior, 35*(3), 239–250.

Franic, T., Kralj, Z., Marcinko, D., Knez, R., & Kardum, G. (2014). Suicidal ideations and sleep-related problems in early adolescence. *Early Intervention in Psychiatry, 8*(2), 155–162. doi:10.1111/eip.12035

Fujino, Y., Mizoue, T., Tokui, N., & Yoshimura, T. (2005). Prospective cohort study of stress, life satisfaction, self-rated health, insomnia, and suicide death in Japan. *Suicide and Life-Threatening Behavior, 35*(2), 227–237. doi:10.1521/suli.35.2.227.62876

Gex, C. R., Narring, F., Ferron, C., & Michaud, P. A. (1998). Suicide attempts among adolescents in Switzerland: Prevalence, associated factors, and comorbidity. *Acta Psychiatrica Scandinavica, 98*, 28–33.

Goetz, R. R., Wolk, S. I., Coplan, J. D., Ryan, N. D., & Weissman, M. M. (2001). Premorbid polysomnographic signs in depressed adolescents: A reanalysis of EEG sleep after long-itudinal follow-up in adulthood. *Biological Psychiatry, 49*, 930–942.

Goldston, D. B., Daniel, S. S., Reboussin, D. M., Reboussin, B. A., Frazier, P. A., & Kelley, A. E. (1999). Suicide attempts among formerly hospitalized adolescents: A prospective naturalistic study of risk during the first five years after discharge. *Journal of the American Academy of Child and Adolescent Psychiatry, 38*(6), 660–671. doi:10.1097/00004583-199906000-00012

Gould, M. S., Marrocco, F. A., Hoagwood, K., Kleinman, M., Amakawa, L., & Altschuler, E. (2009). Service use by at-risk youths after school-based suicide screening. *Journal of the American Academy of Child & Adolescent Psychiatry, 48*(12), 1193–1201. doi:10.1097/CHI.0b013e3181bef6d5

Gregory, A. M., & Sadeh, A. (2016). Annual research review: Sleep problems in childhood psychiatric disorders - a review of the latest science. *The Journal of Child Psychology and Psychiatry, 57*(3), 296–317. doi:10.1111/jcpp.12469

Hayes, A. F. (2013). *Introduction to mediation, moderation, and conditional process analysis: A regression-based approach.* New York, NY: The Guildford Press.

Hill, R. M., Castellanos, D., & Pettit, J. W. (2011). Suicide-related behaviors and anxiety in children and adolescents: A review. *Clinical Psychology Review, 31,* 1133–1144. doi:10.1016/j.cpr.2011.07.008

Hill, R. M., Del Busto, C. T., Buitron, V., & Pettit, J. W. (2018). Depressive symptoms and perceived burdensomeness mediate the association between anxiety and suicidal ideation in adolescents. *Archives of Suicide Research, 22*(4), 555–568. doi:10.1080/13811118.2018.1427163

Iber, C., Ancoli-Israel, S., Chesson, A. L., & Quan, S. F. (2007). The new sleep scoring manual - the evidence behind the rules. *Journal of Clinical Sleep Medicine, 3*(2), 107.

Joiner, T. E. (2005). *Why people die by suicide.* Cambridge, MA: Harvard University Press.

Kelly, R. J., & El-Sheikh, M. (2014). Reciprocal relations between children's sleep and their adjustment over time. *Developmental Psychology, 50*(4), 1137–1147. doi:10.1037/a0034501

Kovacs, M. (1992). *Children's depression inventory.* North Tonawanda, NY: Multi-Health Systems.

Lewis, C. F., Tandon, R., Shipley, J. E., DeQuardo, J. R., Jibson, M., Taylor, S. F., & Goldman, M. (1996). Biological predictors of suicidality in schizophrenia. *Acta Psychiatrica Scandinavica, 94*, 416–420.

Liu, X. (2004). Sleep and adolescent suicidal behavior. *Sleep, 27*(7), 1351–1358. doi:10.1093/sleep/27.7.1351

Liu, X., & Buysse, D. J. (2006). Sleep and youth suicidal behavior: A neglected field. *Current Opinion in Psychiatry, 19*, 288–293. doi:10.1097/01.yco.0000218600.40593.18

Lyneham, H. J., Abbott, M. J., & Rapee, R. M. (2007). Interrater reliability of the anxiety disorders interview schedule for DSM-IV: Child and parent version. *Journal of the American Academy of Child and Adolescent Psychiatry, 46*(6), 731–736. doi:10.1097/chi.0b013e3180465a09

Markovich, A. N., Gendron, M. A., & Corkum, P. V. (2015). Validating the children's sleep habits questionnaire against polysomnography and actigraphy in school-aged children. *Frontiers in Psychology, 5*(188). doi:10.3389/fpsyt.2014.00188

McMakin, D. L., & Alfano, C. A. (2015). Sleep and anxiety in late childhood and early adolescence. *Current Opinion in Psychiatry, 28*(6), 483–489. doi:10.1097/YCO.0000000000000204

Meltzer, L. J., Montgomery-Downs, H. E., Insana, S. P., & Walsh, C. M. (2012). Use of actigraphy for assessment in pediatric sleep research. *Sleep Medicine Reviews, 16*, 463–475. doi:10.1016/j.smrv.2011.10.002

Miklósi, B. J., Kereszténny, M., Hoven, A., Carli, C. W., Wasserman, V., ... Wasserman, D. (2013). Adolescent subthreshold-depression and anxiety: Psychopathology, functional impairment and increased suicide risk. *Journal of Child Psychology and Psychiatry, 54*, 670–677. doi:10.1111/jcpp.12016

Nadorff, M. R., Anestis, M. D., Nazem, S., Harris, H. C., & Winer, E. S. (2014). Sleep disorders and the interpersonal-psychological theory of suicide: Independent pathways to suicidality. *Journal of Affective Disorders, 152*(154), 505–512. doi:10.1016/j.jad.2013.10.011

Noone, D. M., Willis, T. A., Cox, J., Harkness, F., Ogilvie, J., Forbes, E., ... & Gregory, A. M. (2014). Catastrophizing and poor sleep quality in early adolescent females. *Behavioral Sleep Medicine, 12*, 41–52. doi:10.1080/15402002.2013.764528

Owens, J. A., Spirito, A., & McGuinn, M. (2000). The children's sleep habits questionnaire (CSHQ): Psychometric properties of a survey instrument for school-aged children. *Sleep, 23*(8). doi:10.1093/sleep/23.8.1d

Palmer, C. A., & Alfano, C. A. (2017a). Sleep architecture relates to daytime affect and somatic complaints in clinically anxious but not healthy children. *Journal of Clinical Child & Adolescent Psychology, 46*(2), 175–187. doi:10.1080/15374416.2016.1188704

Palmer, C. A., & Alfano, C. A. (2017b). Sleep and emotion regulation: An organizing, integrative review. *Sleep Medicine Reviews, 31*, 6–16. doi:10.1016/j.smrv.2015.12.006

Pigeon, W. R., Pinquart, M., & Conner, K. (2012). Meta-analysis of sleep disturbance and suicidal thoughts and behaviors. *The Journal of Clinical Psychiatry, 73*(9), e1160–e1167. doi:10.4088/JCP.11r07586

Pisani, A. R., Schmeelk-Cone, K., Gunzler, D., Petrova, M., Goldston, D. B., Tu, X., & Wyman, P. A. (2012). Associations between suicidal high school students' help-seeking and their attitudes and perceptions of social environment. *Journal of Youth and Adolescence, 41*, 1312–1324. doi:10.1007/s10964-012-9766-7

Rao, U., Dahl, R. E., Ryan, N. D., Birmaher, B., Williamson, D. E., Giles, D. E., ... Nelson, B. (1996). The relationship between longitudinal clinical course and sleep and cortisol changes in adolescent depression. *Biological Psychiatry, 40*, 474–484. doi:10.1016/0006-3223(95)00481-5

Redfield, R. R., Schuchat, A., Dauphin, L., Cono, J., Richards, C. L., & Iademarco, M. F. (2018). Youth risk behavior surveillance - United States, 2017. *MMWR Surveill Summ, 67*(8), 24–28.

Reinherz, H. Z., Giaconia, R. M., Silverman, A. B., Friedman, A., Pakiz, B., Frost, A. K., & Cohen, E. (1995). Early psychosocial risks for adolescent suicidal ideation and attempts. *Journal of the American Academy of Child and Adolescent Psychiatry, 34*(5), 599–611. doi:10.1097/00004583-199505000-00012

Sabo, E., Reynolds, C. F., III, Kupfer, D. J., & Berman, S. R. (1990). Sleep, depression, and suicide. *Psychiatry Research, 36*, 265–277. doi:10.1016/0165-1781(91)90025-K

Sadeh, A., Sharkey, K. M., & Carskadon, M. A. (1994). Activity-based sleep-wake identification: An empirical test of methodological issues. *Sleep, 17*(3), 201–207. doi:10.1093/sleep/17.3.201

Sareen, J., Cox, B. J., Afifi, T. O., Graaf, R. D., Asmundson, G. J. G., Have, M. T., & Stein, M. B. (2005). Anxiety disorders and risk for suicidal ideation and suicide attempts. *JAMA Psychiatry, 62*, 1249–1257.

Schmeelk-Cone, K., Pisani, A. R., Petrova, M., & Wyman, P. A. (2012). Three scales assessing high school students' attitudes and perceived norms about seeking adult help for distress and suicide concerns. *Suicide and Life-Threatening Behavior, 42*(2), 157–172. doi:10.1111/j.1943-278X.2011.00079.x

Silverman, W. K., & Albano, A. M. (1996). *Anxiety disorders interview schedule for DSM-IV: Parent interview schedule.* San Antonio, TX: Psychological Corporation.

Silverman, W. K., Saavedra, L. M., & Pina, A. A. (2001). Test-retest reliability of anxiety symptoms and diagnoses with the anxiety disorders interview schedule for DSM-IV: Child and parent versions. *Journal of the American Academy of Child and Adolescent Psychiatry*, *40*(8), 937–944. doi:10.1097/00004583-200108000-00016

Tanskanen, A., Tuomilehto, J., Viinamaki, H., Vartiainen, E., Lehtonen, J., & Puska, P. (2001). Nightmares as predictors of suicide. *Sleep*, *24*(7), 845–848. doi:10.1093/sleep/24.7.845

Turvey, C. L., Conwell, Y., Jones, M. P., Phillips, C., Simonsick, E., Pearson, J. L., & Wallace, R. (2002). Risk factors for later-life suicide: A prospective, community-based study. *The American Journal of Geriatric Psychiatry*, *10*(4), 398–406. doi:10.1097/00019442-200207000-00006

Vignau, J., Bailly, D., Duhamel, A., Vervaecke, P., Beuscart, R., & Collinet, C. (1997). Epidemiologic study of sleep quality and troubles in French secondary school adolescents. *Journal of Adolescent Health*, *21*(5), 343–350. doi:10.1016/S1054-139X(97)00109-2

Wechsler, D. (1999). *Manual for the Wechsler abbreviated intelligence scale (WASI)*. San Antonio, TX: The Psychological Corporation.

Weissman, M. M., Wolk, S., Wickramaratne, P., Goldstein, R. B., Adams, P., Greenwald, S.,… Steinberg, D. (1999). Children with prepubertal-onset major depressive disorder and anxiety grown up. *Archives of General Psychiatry*, *56*(9), 794–801. doi:10.1001/archpsyc.56.9.794

Wolk, C. B., Kendall, P. C., & Beidas, R. S. (2015). Cognitive-behavioral therapy for child anxiety confers long-term protection from suicidality. *Journal of the American Academy of Child and Adolescent Psychiatry*, *54*(3), 175–179. doi:10.1016/j.jaac.2014.12.004

Wolk, S. I., & Weissman, M. M. (1996). Suicidal behavior in depressed children grown up: Preliminary results of a longitudinal study. *Psychiatric Annals*, *26*(6), 331–335. doi:10.3928/0048-5713-19960601-11

Wong, M. M., & Brower, K. J. (2012). The prospective relationship between sleep problems and suicidal behavior in the national longitudinal study of adolescent health. *Journal of Psychiatric Research*, *46*(7), 953–959. doi:10.1016/j.jpsychires.2012.04.008

Wong, M. M., Brower, K. J., & Zucker, R. A. (2011). Sleep problems, suicidal ideation, and self-harm behaviors in adolescence. *Journal of Psychiatric Research*, *45*(4), 505–511. doi:10.1016/j.jpsychires.2010.09.005

World Health Organization. (2018). Suicide. Retrieved from http://www.who.int/news-room/fact-sheets/detail/suicide

An examination of the interactive effects of different types of childhood abuse and perceived social support on suicidal ideation

Laura C. Wilson, Amie R. Newins, and Nathan A. Kimbrel

ABSTRACT

No study has examined the interaction between child abuse type and social support in relation to adulthood suicidal ideation. In the present study, 141 female survivors of child sexual abuse or physical abuse completed an online survey of childhood abuse, social support, and suicidal ideation. The findings demonstrated a significant interaction between childhood abuse group and family support, and the interaction between childhood abuse group and friend support approached significance. The present study provides the first evidence that family and friend support may be particularly beneficial in helping to buffer the effects of childhood sexual abuse on risk of adulthood suicidal ideation.

The prevalence of childhood abuse is concerningly high. In a recent study, approximately 12.1% of children experienced at least one form of child abuse (i.e., physical, emotional, or sexual abuse or neglect) in the past year, with 4.0% of children experiencing physical abuse and 2.2% experiencing sexual abuse (Finkelhor, Vanderminden, Turner, Hamby, & Shattuck, 2014). Results of a meta-analysis including studies from 22 different countries revealed that approximately one-fifth (19.7%) of women and one in thirteen (7.9%) men experienced childhood sexual abuse (Pereda, Guilera, Forms, & Gomez-Benito, 2009). Importantly, survivors of child abuse are at increased risk of psychological, behavioral, interpersonal, and physical problems (Briere & Elliott, 2003; Fanslow, Robinson, Crengle, & Perese, 2007; Fergusson, Boden, & Horwood, 2008; Molnar, Buka, & Kessler, 2001; Putnam, 2003). Given the robust relationship between childhood abuse and a range of deleterious outcomes, it is imperative that the field of psychological science work to identify potential areas of intervention that can help improve functioning among survivors.

The rates of suicide within the general population are also alarming. The second leading cause of death among Americans ages 15 to 24 and ages 25 to 34 is suicide; suicide remains in the top 10 leading causes of death among adults between the ages of 55 and 64 (Centers for Disease Control and Prevention, 2015). In a study of individuals ages 15 to 54, between 2.8 and 3.3% reported suicidal ideation in the past 12 months and between 0.7 and 1.0% reported suicide plans (Kessler, Berglund, Borges, Nock, & Wang, 2005). More than one-tenth (11.1%) of college students in one study said they experienced suicidal ideation in the past month and nearly one in six (16.5%) endorsed a history of a suicide attempt (Garlow et al., 2008). Overall, the literature consistently demonstrates high rates of suicidal ideation and attempts, and there is a growing knowledgebase examining factors that impact individuals' risk (e.g., Nock & Kessler, 2006).

Childhood abuse, particularly sexual and physical abuse, is an established risk factor for suicidal ideation and suicide behaviors (Devries et al., 2014; McMahon et al., 2018; Nock & Kessler, 2006). Prior research has demonstrated that survivors of child abuse are four times more likely to attempt suicide in adolescence or adulthood than those who have not experienced childhood abuse (Brown, Cohen, Johnson, & Smailes, 1999). Furthermore, the impact of childhood abuse on mental health persists into later life, even past the age of 60 years (Draper, Pfaff, Pirkis, & Snowdon, 2008). Among the previous studies that have been dedicated to examining explanatory models of suicide, psychopathology is arguably the most studied and consistently demonstrated risk factor (e.g., Nock & Kessler, 2006). Furthermore, because psychopathology (e.g., depression, posttraumatic stress disorder) has been shown to mediate the relationship between childhood adverse events and suicide, the treatment of psychopathology has been suggested as an approach to ameliorate the long-term negative effects of childhood abuse, which includes suicidal ideation (Lopez-Castroman et al., 2015). However, more recent research has demonstrated that childhood abuse has a direct effect on suicide rather than the entirety of the risk being conveyed via psychological disorders (Obikane, Shinozaki, Takagi, & Kawakami, 2018). Therefore, despite a growing literature base that has focused on elucidating the mechanisms that link childhood abuse and suicide, the field still has work to do to better understand the etiology of suicide following childhood abuse.

Although there is a robust direct relationship between childhood abuse and suicidal ideation, not all survivors of child abuse experience suicidal thoughts. Thus, there is a growing literature dedicated to exploring factors that impact child abuse survivors' risk of suicidal ideation, including considering the role of social support (Esposito & Clum, 2002). Social support refers to "the general availability of friends and family members that provide psychological and material resources" (Kleiman & Riskind, 2013, p. 43). Social support has been demonstrated to be a protective factor against the negative effects of childhood abuse, such that social support was negatively associated with anger and depression among women who experienced childhood abuse (Hobfoll et al., 2002). Furthermore, social support has been demonstrated to protect against suicidal ideation and suicidal behaviors in the general population (e.g., Chioqueta & Stiles, 2007; Kleiman & Liu, 2013; Kleiman & Riskind, 2013; Kleiman, Riskind, Schaefer, & Weingarden, 2012).

Several existing studies have examined the role of social support in the relationship between childhood abuse and psychopathology. In one study, there was an interaction between trauma exposure and social support among Kuwaiti girls exposed to war-related trauma such that those who experienced trauma and reported low social support endorsed the highest levels of posttraumatic stress symptoms (Llabre & Hadi, 1997). Among children in foster care, one study found there was a negative relationship between social support and depression symptoms among children who had experienced childhood abuse, and the effect of social support was stronger when children had experienced fewer different types of child abuse (Salazar, Keller, & Courtney, 2011). In a sample of adult women, social support from a friend was protective against depression even after considering the influence of childhood emotional abuse and neglect (Powers, Ressler, & Bradley, 2009). Thus, social support has been supported as one variable that may help the field understand the variability in outcomes observed among childhood abuse survivors.

In one particularly relevant study, Wilson and Scarpa (2014) found a significant interaction between social support from both family and significant others and type of child abuse in relation to posttraumatic stress symptoms in female college students; the interaction between social support from friends and type of child abuse approached statistical significance. Social support from family and friends was protective against posttraumatic stress symptoms among participants who experienced childhood physical abuse but not childhood sexual abuse. Social support from significant others was not related to posttraumatic stress symptoms in survivors of childhood physical abuse, and there was a small positive relationship between support from significant others and posttraumatic stress symptoms among survivors of childhood sexual abuse. In another study, Esposito and Clum (2002) found that the interaction between child sexual abuse and social support satisfaction was significantly related to the severity of suicidal behaviors in a sample of incarcerated adolescents. Specifically, they found that adolescents who experienced severe sexual abuse and reported high social support satisfaction reported lower suicidal ideation than those who experienced severe sexual abuse and low social support satisfaction. The current study aimed to extend the results of the Wilson and Scarpa (2014) and Esposito and Clum (2002) studies by examining whether social support and type of childhood abuse interact to predict adulthood suicidal ideation among women.

Given that previous research has demonstrated that childhood sexual abuse has a stronger relationship with suicide than other forms of childhood abuse (e.g., McMahon et al., 2018), it was hypothesized that survivors of childhood sexual abuse would report higher levels of suicidal ideation. Consistent with prior literature, we also hypothesized that higher levels of social support would be associated with lower levels of suicidal ideation (e.g., Chioqueta & Stiles, 2007; Kleiman & Liu, 2013; Kleiman & Riskind, 2013; Kleiman et al., 2012). Finally, similar to Esposito and Clum (2002), we hypothesized that there would be an interaction between childhood abuse and social support in relation to suicidal ideation.

Method

Participants

The analyzed sample included 141 women who endorsed experiencing either childhood sexual abuse or childhood physical abuse ($M = 24.26$ years, $SD = 10.26$, ranged from 18 to 73 years). The participants were identified through an online survey that was completed by a total of 400 participants. To be included in the analyses, the participants must have also provided complete data for all variables of interest. See Table 1 for more demographic information about the analyzed sample.

Procedure

The data analyzed here were collected as part of a larger 30-minute online survey, which was titled "Childhood experiences and daily life." The Institutional Review Board at the university where the study was conducted approved the study protocol, and each individual participant provided

Table 1. Demographic information for the analyzed sample ($N = 141$).

Variable	n	%	
Race/Ethnicity			
Caucasian/White	100	70.9	
Hispanic/Latino	11	7.8	
African American/Black/African origin	9	6.4	
Asian American/Asian Origin/Pacific Islander	5	3.5	
American Indian/Alaska Native	3	2.1	
Middle Eastern	1	0.7	
Bi-racial/Multi-racial	11	7.8	
Other	1	0.7	
Child Abuse			
Sexual abuse	55	39.0	
Physical abuse only	86	61.0	
	M	SD	Range
Family Social Support	5.40	1.53	1.00–7.00
Friend Social Support	5.71	1.15	1.00–7.00
Significant Other Social Support	6.05	1.17	1.00–7.00
Beck Scale for Suicide Ideation	1.09	1.78	0.00–8.00

informed consent prior to starting the survey. To be included in the larger study, the participants were required to be 18 years of age or older.

Out of the 400 participants who began the survey, 248 signed up through a university psychology subject pool at a small mid-Atlantic public university using an online research management system. After the participants reviewed the informed consent information, they were directed to an anonymous online survey hosted on Qualtrics. Participants from the university psychology subject pool were given course credit toward their introductory psychology course for their participation. The link for the survey was also posted on numerous social media sites (e.g., Facebook, Twitter) that are affiliated with the same university. Therefore, the survey was also open to the public. Of the 400 participants, 152 were recruited through social media. These participants did not receive any incentive for their participation in the study. To protect participants' anonymity, no information was collected related to which participants were recruited through the university psychology subject pool versus social media.

Measures

First, the participants completed a demographic questionnaire that asked them to self-report their age, gender identity, and race/ethnicity. To be included in the present analyses the participants must have reported that their gender identity was female. The current study focused on women because one of the main purposes was to extend the Wilson and Scarpa (2014) study to examine suicidal ideation as the outcome of interest.

Next, participants completed the Childhood Trauma Questionnaire Short Form (CTQ-SF; Bernstein et al., 2003), which was used to identify those who experienced childhood sexual abuse or childhood physical abuse. The CTQ-SF, a 28-item retrospective self-report assessment, asked participants to rate how characteristic each item was of their experiences while they "were growing up." The questionnaire used a 5-point Likert scale (1 = *never true* to 5 = *very often true*). The CTQ-SF contains five subscales (i.e., emotional abuse, physical abuse, sexual abuse, emotional neglect, physical neglect) that each consist of 5-items. The measure also includes three additional items that are used to create a minimization/denial subscale. The sexual abuse (e.g., "Someone tried to make me do sexual things or watch sexual things"), physical abuse (e.g., "People in my family hit me so hard that it left me with bruises or marks"), and minimization/denial (e.g., "I had the perfect childhood") subscales were of interest in the present study. Bernstein et al. (2003) demonstrated that the CTQ-SF has high validity and high reliability. The Cronbach's alphas in the current sample were .84 for the childhood physical abuse subscale and .75 for the childhood sexual abuse subscale, indicating adequate internal consistency.

Participants were identified as having a history of childhood sexual abuse or physical abuse if they responded to at least one relevant item on the corresponding subscales of the CTQ-SF with a response of 2 or greater (i.e., *rarely true* or higher). Conversely, a response of 1 (i.e., *never true*) to all items on a subscale was considered an absence of that type of abuse. Similar to Wilson and Scarpa (2014), if participants reported experiencing both childhood sexual abuse and physical abuse, then they were categorized into the childhood sexual abuse group for the analyses. As noted by Wilson and Scarpa (2014), this procedure was used because childhood sexual abuse often involves physical abuse (e.g., physical force during sexual abuse). This resulted in 86 (61.0%) women who were categorized as having experienced physical abuse and 55 (39.0%) women who were categorized as having experienced sexual abuse. Of the 55 women who endorsed childhood sexual abuse, 38 reported they also experienced childhood physical abuse.

Third, participants completed the Multidimensional Scale of Perceived Social Support (MSPSS; Zimet, Dahlem, Zimet, & Farley, 1988). The MSPSS is a 12-item self-report that assesses three forms of perceived social support, including family support (4 items; e.g., "I could talk about my problems with my family"), friend support (4 items; e.g., "I had friends with whom I could share my joys and sorrows"), and significant other support (4 items; e.g., "There was a romantic partner in my life who cared about my feelings"). The participants responded to each item using a Likert scale ranging from 1 (*very strongly disagree*) to 7 (*very strongly agree*). To calculate the subscale scores, the relevant four items were totaled and divided by four. Higher scores on each subscale were indicative of greater perceived levels of that type of social support. If participants did not have a significant other at the time, then they were instructed to respond *very strongly disagree* for those items because they did not have that source of social support. Prior research has demonstrated adequate reliability and validity for the MSPSS (Dahlem, Zimet, & Walker, 1991). The Cronbach's alphas for the current study were .93 for the family support subscale, .93 for the friend support subscale, and .94 for the significant other support subscale.

Lastly, participants completed the five screening items of the Beck Scale for Suicide Ideation (BSSI; Beck, 1991). This measure assessed the severity of suicidal ideation during the past week, including the day the participants completed the survey. The BSSI uses groups of statements of increasing severity and participants selected the statement that best described them. The scoring for each item ranged from 0 to 2, with greater scores indicating greater suicidal ideation severity. Beck (1991) demonstrated evidence that the BSSI has high reliability and high validity. The Cronbach's alpha in the present study was .82.

Data analysis

All statistical analyses were conducted in SPSS, Version 25. Moderated ordinary least squares (OLS) regression was used to examine the effects of childhood abuse group, perceived social support, and the interaction between childhood abuse group and perceived social support on suicidal ideation. The dichotomous main effect (i.e., childhood abuse group) was dummy coded (i.e., 0 = physical abuse, 1 = sexual abuse) based on recommendations by Dawson (2014). Separate moderation models examined each of the three subscales of the MSPSS (i.e., family support, friend support, significant other support). The CTQ-SF minimization/denial subscale was included as a covariate in all of the moderation models. Prior to conducting the analyses, the continuous moderators and covariate were mean-centered. Each interaction term was created by taking the product of the mean-centered continuous main effect and the binary main effect. When the interaction term was significant, simple slopes were tested according to the procedures recommended by Holmbeck (2002).

Results

Descriptive statistics

Means and standard deviations for continuous variables are presented in Table 1. See Table 2 for the Pearson product moment correlations among the continuous variables of interest. All three forms of perceived social support were significantly positively correlated with each other, which suggests that individuals who perceived high levels of social support from one source tended to perceive high levels of social support from other sources. All three forms of perceived social support were also significantly negatively correlated with suicidal ideation, which indicates that greater perceived social support was associated with lower levels of suicidal ideations. The covariate minimization/denial was significantly positively correlated with family support and significantly negatively correlated with suicidal ideation. An independent samples t-test revealed that although participants who experienced

Table 2. Pearson product moment correlations among the continuous variables of interest.

	1.	2.	3.	4.
1. Family support	-			
2. Friend support	.34**	-		
3. Significant other support	.38**	.29**	-	
4. Suicidal ideation	−.47**	−.28**	−.18*	-
5. Minimization/denial	.22*	.07	.13	−.23*

Note: * $p < .05$, ** $p < .01$.

child sexual abuse and physical abuse did not significantly differ from each other on suicidal ideation (t (86.384) = $-$ 1.56, p = .122), on average, child sexual abuse (M = 1.41, SD = 2.06) was associated with slightly higher levels of suicidal ideation than physical abuse (M = 0.88, SD = 1.55).

Moderation models

The results of the moderation model analyses are presented in Table 3. When examining family support, there was a main effect of family support such that greater family support was associated with lower levels of suicidal ideation. The main effect of childhood abuse group was not significant. There was a significant interaction between childhood abuse group and family support in relation to suicide ideation. Because this interaction was significant, simple slopes analyses were conducted to probe the interaction (see below). When examining friend support, neither the main effect of childhood abuse group nor perceived friend support were significant. Conversely, the interaction between childhood abuse group and friend support approached significance. Although the interaction was not significant, but rather approached significance, the interaction was still probed because moderator effects tend to be small and power may have impacted our ability to detect the interaction (Chaplin, 1991). Finally, when examining significant other support, neither the main effects nor the interaction were significant.

Tests of simple slopes

The simple slopes were examined for the interaction terms involving child abuse type with both family support and friend support. In terms of family

Table 3. Results of ordinary least squares regressions examining childhood abuse group, perceived social support, and the interaction in relation to suicidal ideation.

Model and Predictors	b	SE	β	t
Model 1				
Minimization/denial (covariate)	−.11	.06	−.15	−1.94[a]
Childhood abuse	.31	.28	.08	1.08
Family support	-.32	.13	-.28	-2.54*
Childhood abuse × Family support	-.37	.18	-.22	-2.03*
Model 2				
Minimization/denial (covariate)	−.16	.06	−.23	−2.76**
Childhood abuse	.51	.30	.14	1.70
Friend support	-.17	.18	-.11	-.91
Childhood abuse × Friend support	-.49	.26	-.23	−1.92[a]
Model 3				
Minimization/denial (covariate)	−.15	.06	−.21	−2.44*
Childhood abuse	.52	.31	.14	1.66
Significant other support	-.18	.17	-.12	−1.11
Childhood abuse × Significant other support	-.12	.27	-.05	-.45

Notes. Childhood abuse (0 = physical abuse; 1 = sexual abuse); **p < .01, *p < .05, [a]p < .06.

support, these analyses indicated that the effect of perceived family support on suicidal ideation was significant for both the physical abuse group ($b = - .32$, $SE = .13$, $\beta = - .28$, $t = - 2.54$, $p = .012$) and the sexual abuse group ($b = - .69$, $SE = .13$, $\beta = - .60$, $t = - 5.20$, $p < .001$; See Figure 1), although the effects differed in magnitude. In terms of friend support, these analyses indicated that the effect of friend support on suicidal ideation was not significant for the physical abuse group ($b = - .17$, $SE = .18$, $\beta = - .11$, $t = - .91$, $p = .37$) but was significant for the sexual abuse group ($b = - .66$, $SE = .18$, $\beta = - .42$, $t = - 3.65$, $p < .001$; See Figure 2).

Discussion

The objective of the present study was to extend the prior work of Wilson and Scarpa (2014) and Esposito and Clum (2002), both of which examined the interaction between social support and childhood abuse in relation to mental health outcomes. Surprisingly, in the present study, the independent samples t-test and main effects in the moderated OLS regression revealed there was no significant bivariate relationship between childhood abuse type and suicidal ideation. We had hypothesized that survivors of childhood sexual abuse would report significantly higher levels of suicidal ideation than survivors of physical abuse only. This hypothesis was consistent with a number of prior studies that have demonstrated a stronger association between sexual abuse and suicidal behavior than among survivors of other types of childhood abuse (e.g., McMahon et al., 2018). The present study demonstrated that the relationship between child abuse type and suicidal

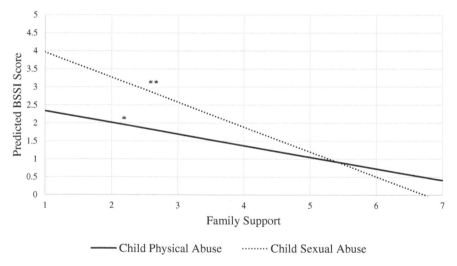

Figure 1. Graph of the interaction between childhood abuse group and levels of perceived family support. *indicates significant simple slope at $p < .05$,
** indicates significant simple slope at $p < .001$.

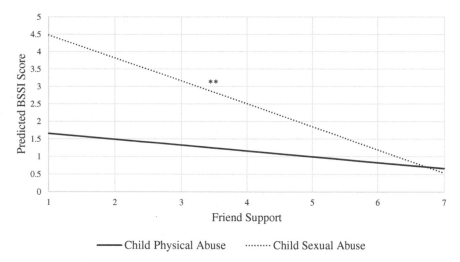

Figure 2. Graph of the interaction between childhood abuse group and levels of perceived friend support.
**indicates significant simple slope at $p < .001$.

ideation may in fact be more complicated. Specifically, the significant inter-action between child abuse type and social support in relation to suicidal ideation supports that it would be ill-advised to examine the main effect of abuse type on suicidal ideation.

The present study found evidence to support our hypothesis that higher levels of social support would be associated with lower levels of suicidal ideation. Specifically, we observed negative bivariate associations between suicidal ideation and each of the three forms of social support we measured, which included social support from family members, friends, and significant others. This finding is consistent with prior research demonstrating that increased social support may be protective against suicidal ideation and suicide attempts (e.g., Carpenter et al., 2015; DeBeer, Kimbrel, Meyer, Gulliver, & Morissette, 2014; Kleiman & Liu, 2013), including Kleiman and Liu (2013) who found that social support was associated with decreased risk for suicide attempts in two large nationally representative samples after accounting for a number of important covariates.

Finally, the current study significantly adds to the field's understanding of the complexity of the association between different forms of childhood abuse and social support in relation to suicidal ideation by demonstrating for the first time that different types of social support can potentially moderate the impact of childhood abuse on risk for adulthood suicidal ideation. Specifically, the present study builds on Esposito and Clum (2002), which focused on childhood abuse and social support in relation to suicidal ideation among adolescents who were juvenile delinquents. The present study demonstrated that family and friend support may be particularly beneficial in helping to buffer the effects of childhood sexual abuse on adult survivors' risk for suicidal ideation, as we observed that lower levels of perceived social support from family and friends were more strongly associated with higher levels of suicidal ideation among survivors of childhood sexual abuse relative to survivors of childhood physical abuse. While these results are clearly in need of replication, they indicate that women who experienced childhood sexual abuse may be especially likely to benefit from interventions aimed at increasing their perceived social support from friends and family members. This result is consistent with Esposito and Clum (2002), who also found that the impact of social support on suicidal ideation was stronger among sexual abuse survivors than physical abuse survivors. Esposito and Clum argued that it is possible that physical abuse survivors may be less likely to look to others for support in coping with their victimization experiences, and this explanation may hold true for our results as well.

While it is unclear at the present time why perceived social support from significant others was unrelated to suicidal ideation in the regression analyses, one potential explanation is that committed romantic relationships may have been less common and more unstable in this sample, since the majority of the participants were college students who were well below the average age of marriage for women, which is currently estimated to be 27.4 years of age by the U.S. Census Bureau (2018). Thus, it is possible that the potential impact of perceived social support from significant others could increase as women age and become involved in more stable and long-term relationships, whereas the role of social support from friends and family could potentially diminish. While the present study is unable to speak to this question directly, it is noteworthy that a 2018 meta-analysis by Kyung-Sook, SangSoo, Sangjin, and Young-Jeon that included millions of participants found that marriage conveyed a protective effect against suicide, such that non-married individuals' multivariate-adjusted risk for suicide was 92% higher (i.e., AOR = 1.92) than the risk observed among married individuals, after adjusting for a variety of covariates. Thus, a particularly important future direction for this work would be to conduct a prospective study aimed at understanding if and how the interactive effects between social support and child abuse might change over time.

Study limitations

The findings from the present study should be interpreted within the context of several important limitations. First, the present study included a convenience sample of women who were recruited from a university and through social media. Thus, it is impossible to know the degree to which the findings might generalize to the larger population of U.S. women, but the demographic characteristics of the sample (e.g., race/ethnicity) were consistent with the university used for recruitment. Second, the study was cross-sectional in nature and the measurements of childhood abuse were retrospective in nature. While we did use a well-known and well-validated measure of childhood abuse to overcome the latter issue, it is impossible to rule out recall bias. Third, we are unable to infer causality in the present study due to the cross-sectional design. Furthermore, because the MSPSS assessed current social support and the BSSI assessed suicidal ideation in the past week, we were unable to consider the influence of past levels of social support or suicidality. Future researchers should use a longitudinal design which would allow them to better establish the temporal order of the variables, assess the variables of interest at multiple time points, and account for additional relevant factors (e.g., prior psychotherapy, more recent traumatic events). This is particularly noteworthy given that prior research has demonstrated that social support may mediate the relationship between childhood abuse and mental health outcomes (Sperry & Widom, 2013). Fourth, because our study was restricted to women, the degree to which these findings might generalize to individuals of other genders (e.g., individuals who identify as men or non-binary) is unknown and should be a focus of future research. Finally, the present study did not consider the influence of other potentially relevant variables, such as age, education, or gender (Angst et al., 2014; Obikane et al., 2018). For example, prior research has demonstrated that low social support is a stronger risk factor for suicidal ideation among women and sexual abuse is a stronger risk factor for suicidal ideation among men (Angst et al., 2014). Therefore, future researchers should consider whether the buffering effect of social support on the relationship between childhood abuse and suicidal ideation is impacted by other variables.

Implications for practice

The present findings have a number of important implications for clinical practice. Our findings provide evidence that childhood sexual abuse is a significant risk factor for suicidal ideation, particularly among those with low levels of family and friend support. As such, clinicians working with survivors of childhood sexual abuse should routinely assess for suicidal ideation and, when indicated, intervene to reduce patients' risk for suicide attempts. There are now a number of promising interventions aimed at decreasing the occurrence of suicidal behavior among high-risk patients, including Stanley and Brown (2012) Safety Planning Intervention, which was recently found to reduce the occurrence of suicidal behaviors among suicidal patients by approximately half over a period of six months (Stanley et al., 2018).

The present findings also suggest that survivors of childhood sexual abuse may be especially likely to benefit from interventions aimed at increasing their perceived social support from friends and family members. Indeed, when social support from family and friends was perceived to be high, severity of suicidal ideation was markedly lower among survivors of childhood sexual abuse and was quite similar to the magnitude observed among survivors of childhood physical abuse (see Figures 1 and 2). Thus, in addition to providing evidence-based treatment for any psychological disorders (e.g., PTSD, depression) stemming from the abuse, the present findings indicate that clinicians may also want to work with patients to find ways to enhance their perceived social support from family members and existing friends and peers. Clinicians might also want to consider recommending that patients become involved in peer support groups for survivors of childhood sexual abuse to further augment their ongoing evidence-based treatment.

In sum, the findings from the present study provide further evidence that higher levels of perceived social support are associated with decreased risk for suicidal ideation. Moreover, the results supported an interaction between perceived social support and childhood abuse that suggests that survivors of childhood sexual abuse may be especially likely to benefit from interventions aimed at increasing perceived social support from family and friends as a mechanism for reducing risk for suicidal ideation during adulthood. Further work on this topic would benefit from the use of longitudinal designs, as well as more diverse and representative samples.

Disclosure statement

No potential conflict of interest was reported by the authors.

References

Angst, J., Hengartner, M. P., Rogers, J., Schnyder, U., Steinhausen, H. C., Ajdacic-Gross, V., & Rossler, W. (2014). Suicidality in the prospective Zurich study: Prevalence, risk factors and gender. *European Archives of Psychiatry and Clinical Neuroscience, 264,* 557–565. doi:10.1007/s00406-014-0500-1

Beck, A. T. (1991). *Beck scale for suicide ideation: Manual.* New York, NY: The Psychological Corporation.

Bernstein, D. P., Stein, J. S., Newcomb, M. D., Walker, E., Pogge, D., Ahluvalia, T., ... Zule, W. (2003). Development and validation of a brief screening version of the Childhood Trauma Questionnaire. *Child Abuse & Neglect, 27,* 169–190. doi:10.1016/S0145-2134(02)00541-0

Briere, J., & Elliott, D. M. (2003). Prevalence and psychological sequelae of self-report childhood physical and sexual abuse in a general population sample of men and women. *Child Abuse & Neglect, 27,* 1205–1222. doi:10.1016/j.chiabu.2003.09.008

Brown, J., Cohen, P., Johnson, J. G., & Smailes, E. M. (1999). Childhood abuse and neglect: Specificity of effects on adolescent and young adult depression and suicidality. *Journal of the American Academy of Child & Adolescent Psychiatry, 38,* 1490–1496. doi:10.1097/00004583-199912000-00009

Carpenter, G. S. J., Carpenter, T. P., Kimbrel, N. A., Flynn, E. J., Pennington, M. L., Cammarata, C., ... Gulliver, S. B. (2015). Social support, stress, and suicidal ideation among professional firefighters. *American Journal of Health Behavior, 39*(2), 191–196. PMID: 25564831. doi:10.5993/AJHB.39.2.5

Center for Disease Control and Prevention. (2015). *10 leading causes of death by age group, United States – 2015.* Retrieved from https://www.cdc.gov/injury/images/lc-charts/leading_causes_of_death_age_group_2015_1050w740h.gif

Chaplin, W. F. (1991). The next generation of moderator research in personality psychology. *Journal of Personality, 59,* 143–178. doi:10.1111/j.1467-6494.1991.tb00772.x

Chioqueta, A. P., & Stiles, T. C. (2007). The relationship between psychological buffers, hopelessness, and suicidal ideation: Identification of protective factors. *Crisis, 28,* 67–73. doi:10.1027/0227-5910.28.2.67

Dahlem, N. W., Zimet, G. D., & Walker, R. R. (1991). The multidimensional scale of perceived social support: A confirmation study. *Journal of Clinical Psychology, 47,* 756–761. doi:10.1002/1097-4679(199111)47:6

Dawson, J. F. (2014). Moderation in management research: What, why, when, and how. *Journal of Business and Psychology, 29,* 1–19. doi:10.1007/s10869-013-9308-7

DeBeer, B. B., Kimbrel, N. A., Meyer, E. C., Gulliver, S. B., & Morissette, S. B. (2014). Combined posttraumatic (PTSD) and depressive symptoms interact with social support to predict suicidal ideation in Operation Enduring Freedom and Operation Iraqi Freedom (OEF/OIF) veterans. *Psychiatry Research, 216,* 357–362. PMID: 25612971. doi:10.1016/j.psychres.2014.02.010

Devries, K. M., Mak, J. Y. T., Child, J. C., Falder, G., Bacchus, L. J., Astbury, J., & Watts, C. H. (2014). Childhood sexual abuse and suicidal behavior: A meta-analysis. *Pediatrics, 135,* e1331–e1344. doi:10.1542/peds.2013-2166

Draper, B., Pfaff, J. J., Pirkis, J., & Snowdon, J. (2008). Long-term effects of childhood abuse on the quality of life and health of older people: Results from the depression and early prevention of suicide in general practice project. *Journal of the American Geriatrics Society, 56,* 262–271. doi:10.1111/j.1532-5415.2007.01537.x

Esposito, C. L., & Clum, G. A. (2002). Social support and problem-solving as moderators of the relationship between childhood abuse and suicidality: Applications to a delinquent population. *Journal of Traumatic Stress, 15,* 137–146. doi:10.1023/A:1014860024980

Fanslow, J. L., Robinson, E. M., Crengle, S., & Perese, L. (2007). Prevalence of child sexual abuse reported by cross-sectional sample of New Zealand women. *Child Abuse & Neglect, 31,* 935–945. doi:10.1016/j.chiabu.2007.02.009

Fergusson, D. M., Boden, J. M., & Horwood, L. J. (2008). Exposure to childhood sexual and physical abuse and adjustment in early adulthood. *Child Abuse & Neglect, 32,* 607–619. doi:10.1016/j.chiabu.2006.12.018

Finkelhor, D., Vanderminden, J., Turner, H., Hamby, S., & Shattuck, A. (2014). Child maltreatment rates assessed in a national household survey of caregivers and youth. *Child Abuse & Neglect, 38,* 1421–1435. doi:10.1016/j.chiabu.2014.05.005

Garlow, S. J., Rosenberg, J., Moore, J. D., Haas, A. P., Koestner, B., Hendin, H., & Nemeroff, C. B. (2008). Depression, desperation, and suicidal ideation in college students: Results from the American foundation for suicide prevention college screening project at emory university. *Depression and Anxiety, 25,* 482–488. doi:10.1002/da.20321

Hobfoll, S. E., Bansal, A., Schurg, R., Young, S., Pierce, C. A., Hobfoll, I., & Johnson, R. (2002). The impact of perceived child physical and sexual abuse history on Native American women's psychological well-being and AIDS risk. *Journal of Consulting and Clinical Psychology, 70,* 252–257. doi:10.1037/0022-006X.70.1.252

Holmbeck, G. N. (2002). Post-hoc probing of significant moderational and mediational effects in studies on pediatric populations. *Journal of Pediatric Psychology, 27,* 87–96. doi:10.1093/jpepsy/27.1.87

Kessler, R. C., Berglund, P., Borges, G., Nock, M., & Wang, P. S. (2005). Trends in suicide ideation, plans, gestures, and attempts in the United States, 1990-1992 to 2001-2003. *Journal of the American Medical Association, 293,* 2487–2495. doi:10.1001/jama.293.20.2487

Kleiman, E. M., & Liu, R. T. (2013). Social support as a protective factor in suicide: Findings from two nationally representative samples. *Journal of Affective Disorders, 150,* 540–545. doi:10.1016/j.jad.2013.01.033

Kleiman, E. M., & Riskind, J. H. (2013). Utilized social support and self-esteem mediate the relationship between perceived social support and suicide ideation: A test of a multiple mediator model. *Crisis, 34,* 42–49. doi:10.1027/0227-5910/a00159

Kleiman, E. M., Riskind, J. H., Schaefer, K. E., & Weingarden, H. (2012). The moderating role of social support on the relationship between impulsivity and suicide risk. *Crisis, 33,* 273–279. doi:10.1027/0227-5910/a000136

Kyung-Sook, W., SangSoo, S., Sangjin, S., & Young-Jeon, S. (2018). Marital status integration and suicide: A meta-analysis and meta-regression. *Social Science & Medicine, 197,* 116–126. doi:10.1016/j.socscimed.2017.11.053

Llabre, M. M., & Hadi, F. (1997). Social support and psychological distress in Kuwaiti boys and girls exposed to the Gulf crisis. *Journal of Clinical Child Psychology, 26,* 247–255. doi:10.1207/s15374424jccp2603_3

Lopez-Castroman, J., Jaussent, I., Beziat, S., Guillaume, S., Baca-Garcia, E., Olie, E., & Courtet, P. (2015). Posttraumatic stress disorder following childhood abuse increases the severity of suicide attempts. *Journal of Affective Disorders, 170,* 7–14. doi:10.1016/j.jad.2014.08.010

McMahon, K., Hoertel, N., Olfson, M., Wall, M., Wang, S., & Blanco, C. (2018). Childhood maltreatment and impulsivity as predictors of interpersonal violence, self-injury and suicide attempts: A national study. *Psychiatry Research, 26i,* 386–393. doi:10.1016/j.psychres.2018.08.059

Molnar, B. E., Buka, S. L., & Kessler, R. C. (2001). Childhood sexual abuse and subsequent psychopathology: Results from the national comorbidity survey. *American Journal of Public Health, 91,* 753–760. doi:10.2105/AJPH.91.5.753

Nock, M. K., & Kessler, R. C. (2006). Prevalence of and risk factors for suicide attempts versus suicide gestures: Analysis of the national comorbidity study. *Journal of Abnormal Psychology, 115,* 616–623. doi:10.1037/0021-843X.115.3.616

Obikane, E., Shinozaki, T., Takagi, D., & Kawakami, N. (2018). Impact of childhood abuse on suicide-related behavior. Analysis using structural models. *Journal of Affective Disorders, 234,* 224–230. doi:10.1016/j.jad.2018.02.034

Pereda, N., Guilera, G., Forms, M., & Gomez-Benito, J. (2009). The prevalence of child sexual abuse in community and study samples: A meta-analysis. *Clinical Psychology Review, 29,* 328–338. doi:10.1016/j.cpr.2009.02.007

Powers, A., Ressler, K. J., & Bradley, R. G. (2009). The protective role of friendship on effects of childhood abuse and depression. *Depression and Anxiety, 26,* 45–53. doi:10.1002/da.20534

Putnam, F. W. (2003). Ten-year research update review: Child sexual abuse. *Journal of the American Academy of Child and Adolescent Psychiatry, 42,* 269–278. doi:10.1097/00004583-200303000-00006

Salazar, A. M., Keller, T. E., & Courtney, M. E. (2011). Understanding social support's role in the relationship between maltreatment and depression in youth with foster care experience. *Child Maltreatment, 16,* 102–113. doi:10.1177/1077559511402985

Sperry, D. M., & Widom, C. S. (2013). Child abuse and neglect, social support, and psychopathology in adulthood: A prospective investigation. *Child Abuse & Neglect, 37,* 415–425. doi:10.1016/j.chiabu.2013.02.006

Stanley, B., & Brown, G. K. (2012). Safety planning intervention: A brief intervention to mitigate suicide risk. *Cognitive and Behavioral Practice, 19,* 256–264. doi:10.1016/j.cbpra.2011.01.001

Stanley, B., Brown, G. K., Brenner, L. A., Galfvalvy, H. C., Currier, G. W., Knox, K. L., … Green, K. L. (2018). Comparison of the safety planning intervention with follow-up vs usual care of suicidal patients treated in the emergency eepartment. *JAMA Psychiatry, 75* (9), 894–900. doi:10.1001/jamapsychiatry.2018.1776

U.S. Census Bureau. (2018). *Historical marital status tables.* Retrieved from https://www.census.gov/data/tables/time-series/demo/families/marital.html

Wilson, L. C., & Scarpa, A. (2014). Childhood abuse, perceived social support, and posttraumatic stress symptoms: A moderation model. *Psychological Trauma: Theory, Research, Practice, and Policy, 6,* 512–518. doi:10.1037/a0032635

Zimet, G. D., Dahlem, N. W., Zimet, S. G., & Farley, G. K. (1988). The multidimensional scale of perceived social support. *Journal of Personality Assessment, 52,* 30–41. doi:10.1207/s15327752jpa5201_2

Violent victimization and perpetration as distinct risk factors for adolescent suicide attempts

Evan E. Rooney (ID), Ryan M. Hill, Benjamin Oosterhoff, and Julie B. Kaplow

ABSTRACT

This study examined associations among violent victimization, perpetration, and suicide attempts in youth reporting suicide ideation, within an ideation-to-action framework of suicide. Data on 821 youth (Mage = 16.20, SD = 1.66) were drawn from the National Longitudinal Study of Adolescent to Adult Health, with information regarding violent victimization and perpetration, history of suicide ideation and attempts, non-violent delinquency, depressive symptoms, and substance use. Hierarchical regression analyses indicated that greater experiences of violent victimization and the interaction of violence perpetration by victimization were associated with greater frequency of suicide attempts. Consistent with an ideation-to-action framework, results indicate that violent experiences (victimization or perpetration) may increase the capability for suicide.

Suicide is the second leading cause of death for adolescents and young adults in the United States (Centers for Disease Control and Prevention, 2018a), and suicide-related behaviors are a serious public health concern. Adolescence appears to be a crucial period for the onset of suicide-related behaviors: The suicide rate increases from 0.29 per 100,000 children at age 10 to 17.32 per 100,000 by age 21 and remains elevated throughout adulthood (CDC, 2018a). Although the rate of suicide increases dramatically across adolescence, the rate of suicide ideation remains relatively high across middle school and high school youth; 16% – 25% of middle school youth and 17% of high school youth report seriously considering suicide in the previous 12 months (Centers for Disease Control and Prevention, 2018b; Kann et al., 2018). The increase in suicide deaths, coupled with steady suicide ideation rates, suggests that adolescence may be a key period of onset for factors associated with the transition from suicide ideation to suicide behavior. Understanding factors that promote this transition is a crucial goal for suicide research, as only a subset of those who consider suicide actually act on their suicidal thoughts (Kessler, Borges, & Walters, 1999; Nock et al., 2008; Ten Have et al., 2009).

However, relatively little work has examined risk factors specific to suicide attempts (May & Klonsky, 2016).

Exposure to violence through victimization and acts of perpetration may contribute to risk for suicide attempts during adolescence. Violent victimization and perpetration increase during adolescence (Finkelhor, Turner, Ormrod, & Hamby, 2009; Moffitt, 1993), and experiencing violent victimization and perpetration may provide youth with the capability (e.g., fearlessness, physical means) for suicide behavior. The current study examined the potential associations between violent victimization, perpetration, and suicide attempts among a national sample of youth endorsing suicide ideation.

Ideation-to-action theories of suicide

Several recent theories of suicide-related behavior propose an "ideation-to-action" framework, in which suicide ideation and suicide attempts have distinct risk markers and causal processes (Klonsky & May, 2015; O'Connor, 2011; Van Orden et al., 2010). While there is considerable evidence supporting the associations between various risk factors (e.g., depression, hopelessness, social isolation, and negative life events) and suicide *ideation* (see Van Orden et al., 2010 for a review), comparatively less work has focused on identifying risk factors specific to suicide *behavior* (May & Klonsky, 2016). Identification of factors associated with the transition from ideation to action is key for identifying potential mechanisms for intervention and improving suicide prevention efforts (Fergusson, Beautrais, & Horwood, 2003; Kessler et al., 1999; Nock et al., 2008; Ten Have et al., 2009).

One such ideation-to-action theory is the interpersonal-psychological theory of suicide (IPTS; Joiner, 2005; Van Orden et al., 2010). The IPTS proposes that suicide ideation occurs in the joint presence of two proximal risk factors, thwarted belongingness and perceived burdensomeness (Joiner, 2005), and a substantial evidence base supports this hypothesis among adolescent samples (for reviews, see Hill & Pettit, 2014; Stewart, Eaddy, Horton, Hughes, & Kennard, 2017). Under the IPTS framework, the transition from suicide ideation to serious suicide behaviors requires the acquired capability to enact lethal self-injury (Joiner, 2005). This acquired capability, attained via exposure to painful and provocative events, is hypothesized to result from increased fearlessness about death and pain tolerance (Van Orden et al., 2010). Evidence from a variety of samples supports the hypothesis that the acquired capability is associated with increased rates of serious suicide behavior (Anestis, Khazem, Mohn, & Green, 2015; Czyz, Berona, & King, 2015; Van Orden et al., 2010).

Another ideation-to-action theory is the integrated motivational-volitional model of suicide behavior (IMV; O'Connor, 2011). The IMV consists of three phases: the pre-motivational phase (i.e., predisposition towards suicide including individual differences and negative life experiences), the motivational phase (i.e., formation of suicide ideation), and the volitional phase (i.e., formation of the capability for suicide). The motivational phase is denoted by feelings of defeat, humiliation, and entrapment, which have been associated with suicide ideation (Dhingra, Boduszek, & O'Connor, 2015, 2016). The volitional phase represents the shift from suicide ideation to suicide behavior and is hypothesized to include factors such as capability, impulsivity, and access to means (O'Connor, 2011). Unlike the IPTS, the IMV takes into account a broader range of genetic and personality factors as direct (versus indirect) contributors to the volitional shift from suicide ideation to suicide attempts. Research has also demonstrated that this set of factors is associated with suicide attempts (Dhingra et al., 2015).

A third ideation-to-action model is the Three-Step Theory (3ST; Klonsky & May, 2015). The 3ST posits that suicide ideation develops in the presence of day-to-day experiences of pain (e.g., emotional pain, physical pain, social isolation) paired with a sense of hopelessness about the future. The second step, following every day experiences of pain, is the development of serious or active ideation, which forms when an individual's pain becomes greater than their connectedness. Finally, like other ideation-to-action models, the 3ST emphasizes the capability for suicide as a necessary component for suicide behavior with the intent to die. Klonsky and May (2015) highlight a range of factors that contribute to the development of this capability, including: dispositional (i.e., inherited genetic or temperamental traits), acquired (e.g., exposure to events that habituate one to experiences of fear, pain, or death), and practical (e.g., access to firearms) factors. Initial empirical studies support the hypotheses of the 3ST (Dhingra, Klonsky, & Tapola, 2018; May & Klonsky, 2016).

Common across these ideation-to-action models, the transition from suicide ideation to suicide behavior requires the development of the capability for suicide, characterized by habituation to the innate fear of death evoked by suicide ideation. The elucidation of specific factors or experiences associated with suicide behavior may provide greater insight into the development of suicide capability and help identify potential mechanisms for suicide prevention and intervention. Consistent with the theories outlined above, the present study aims to elucidate risk markers that may be important for the conceptually distinct process of engaging in suicide attempts by only testing our models among participants who have reported experiencing suicide ideation. Specifically, we propose two risk factors for suicide attempts that may contribute to the capability for suicide among those experiencing suicide ideation: violence victimization and violence perpetration.

Risk factors for suicide attempts: The role of violent victimization and perpetration

Adolescent experiences with violence through victimization and perpetration, insofar as these experiences may involve substantial exposure to pain or risk of physical injury, represent candidate mechanisms for developing the acquired capability and increasing the likelihood of engaging in suicide behavior. Interpersonal violence exposure is associated with suicide attempts and suicide among youth and young adults (Castellví et al., 2017). Additionally, in a population-based survey of U.S. adults, those who experienced violent victimization at the hands of police officers had a significantly increased likelihood of suicide attempts than those who did not (DeVylder et al., 2017). These data suggest the importance of violent victimization as a factor associated with suicide behavior. Within ideation-to-action frameworks, experiences characterized by traumatic victimization may serve to increase suicide capability through habituation to the fear of death or increased pain tolerance.

Violence exposure may also take the form of perpetration, and those who perpetrate violent acts may also experience habituation to fear of death and thus acquire suicide capability. Engaging in violence during adolescence is associated with both suicide ideation and attempts in young adulthood (Van Dulmen et al., 2013), and conduct disorder is associated with suicide attempts among adults with suicide ideation, even after adjusting for other psychiatric disorders (Borges, Nock, Medina-Mora, Hwang, & Kessler, 2010). Evidence also links bully perpetration to youth suicide-related behaviors (Arango, Opperman, Gipson, & King, 2016; Klomek et al., 2013; Thomas et al., 2017). Among adults, those who perpetrate violence are more likely to report suicide attempts (Ilgen et al., 2010). Taken together, this research highlights the potential role of adolescent violence perpetration as a risk marker for suicide attempts, in addition to violent victimization.

While both violent victimization and perpetration are associated with suicide behavior generally, little research has investigated suicide behaviors among those who are both victims and perpetrators. For example, research examining suicide risk among bully-victims (i.e., those who bully others and are bullied themselves) suggests that they are at greater risk for suicide than those who are only victims *or* perpetrators (Hepburn, Azrael, Molnar, & Miller, 2012; Kiriakidis, 2008; Klomek, Marrocco, Kleinman, Schonfeld, & Gould, 2007). Within ideation-to-action frameworks, the combination of violence victimization and perpetration may indicate a high degree of suicide capability and therefore be strongly associated with suicide attempts. Thus, it is important to determine whether those who both experience and perpetrate violence are at greater risk for engaging in suicide behaviors, and whether this effect is additive (independent main effects) or multiplicative (interactive effects). Little research has explicitly examined the independent and interactive effects of violent victimization and perpetration on suicide attempts among adolescents who report suicide ideation. Testing these associations may help elucidate the potential role of violence exposure in promoting adolescent suicide behaviors and provide novel insight into developmental processes that potentially contribute to increased suicide attempts during this age period.

Current study

The present study examined the associations between violent victimization and perpetration and suicide attempts, among those who endorsed suicide ideation in the past year, in a national sample of youth. Focusing only on those who endorsed suicide ideation enables the analyses to examine factors associated with suicide attempts after controlling for the presence of suicide ideation. That is, this approach allows for the examination of factors associated with the transition from suicide ideation to suicide attempt, by limiting analyses to only those with suicide ideation. We hypothesized that violent victimization and perpetration would be associated with more frequent suicide attempts made during the past year. Based on prior research on adolescent bully-victims (Hepburn et al., 2012; Kiriakidis, 2008; Klomek et al., 2007), we also expected that that the effects of victimization on suicide attempts would be stronger for youth who report higher violence perpetration. To further clarify the role of violence perpetration, analyses accounted for demographic characteristics, depressive symptoms, non-violent delinquency, and substance use. Depressive symptoms were included as they are strongly associated with victimization (Deeds, Lagrange, Simoni-Wastila, & Peralta, 2007; Kimmel, 2014) and suicidality (Van Orden et al., 2010) and their inclusion enabled us to examine the role of violence exposure beyond that of an established predictive factor for suicidality. Non-violent delinquency and substance use were also included as they may indicate painful or provocative experiences and enabled us to contrast the role of violence perpetration with other externalizing behaviors (see May & Victor, 2018 for a review).

Method

Participants

Data were drawn from the National Longitudinal Study of Adolescent to Adult Health (Add Health) database. Details regarding the Add Health database are available elsewhere (Harris, 2013; Resnick et al., 1997). This study utilizes Wave 1 (1994–1995) of the public use dataset, which included responses for $n = 6,054$ adolescents ($M_{age} = 16.09$, SD = 1.61, range: 13–21). Of the youth who completed Wave 1 of the Add Health study, $n = 821$ indicated that they had seriously thought about committing suicide in the past year and these youth comprised the analytic sample. Participants (63.1% female; $M_{age} = 16.20$, SD = 1.66, range: 13–21) were primarily White (64.7%), African American/Black (16.8%), Asian (3.9%), Native American (1.7%), other (6.4%), or biracial (6.5%) and 12.1% of participants identified as Hispanic. The median household income was $40,000 (range: $0 – $900,000). Regarding parent education, 15.8% of parent respondents (16.0% of spouses) did not complete high school, 38.9% completed high school without college training (40.9% spouses), 19.3% completed some college (16.4% spouses), and 25.9% obtained a college degree or higher (26.7% of spouses).

Measures

Suicide attempts

Participants' history of suicide attempts was measured using one item that assessed the frequency with which youth attempted suicide in the last 12 months. Responses were given using a 5-point scale ranging from 0 (*0 times*) to 4 (*6 or more times*).

Violent victimization

Consistent with prior research (Oosterhoff, Kaplow, & Layne, 2016), participants reported the number of times they were exposed to six types of violent events during the past 12 months. These events included witnessing a shooting/stabbing, being held at knife/gunpoint, being shot, being stabbed, being jumped, or being in a physical fight that resulted in a serious injury. Responses were given on a 3-point scale comprised of 0 (*never*), 1 (*once*), and 2 (*more than once*). Mean scores were created with higher values indicating greater violence exposure (α = .75).

Violence perpetration

Violence perpetration was measured with two items (r = .31) assessing the frequency with which youth had seriously injured someone or used or threatened someone with a weapon in the past 12 months. Responses were given on a 3-point scale comprised of 0 (*never*), 1 (*once*), and 2 (*more than once*). Mean scores were created with higher values indicating greater violence perpetration (α = .60).

Non-violent delinquency

Non-violent delinquency was measured with 10 items assessing the frequency with which youth had engaged in various forms of delinquent behavior (i.e., paint graffiti, damage property, lie to parents, run away from home, steal a car, sell drugs, burglarize a building, shoplift, steal property valued over $50, steal property valued under $50) in the past 12 months. Responses were given on a 3-point scale comprised of 0 (*never*), 1 (*once*), and 2 (*more than once*). Mean scores were created with higher values indicating greater non-violent delinquency (α = .80).

Binge drinking and marijuana use

Substance use was measured using two items assessing adolescents' frequency of binge drinking and marijuana use. Binge drinking was measured via a single item assessing the frequency youth had gotten drunk in the past 12 months. Responses were given on a 7-point scale from 1 (*never*) to 7 (*everyday*). Marijuana use was measured using a single item assessing the frequency youth had used marijuana or hashish in the past 30 days. Responses were given in count format. Items were modeled separately because of the different response scaling with higher values indicating greater binge drinking and marijuana use.

Depressive symptoms

Depressive symptoms were measured with the 20-item version of the Center for Epidemiologic Studies Depression Scale (CESD-20; Hann, Winter, & Jacobsen, 1999). Participants rated their agreement with 20 statements about how they have felt in the past 7 days (e.g., feeling bothered by things) on a 4-point scale ranging from 0 (*never/rarely*) to 3 (*most/all of the time*). Mean scores were calculated with higher values indicating more depressive symptoms ($\alpha = .91$).

Demographics

Participants reported their date of birth which was used to compute age at time of assessment. Participants were also asked to report their ethnicity (i.e., Hispanic or non-Hispanic) and their race (i.e., White, Black or African-American, American Indian or Native American, Asian or Pacific Islander, or Other). Additionally, participants' parents reported their household income; ratio of the federal poverty line was calculated from this value and was used for all analyses.

Analytic technique

Stepwise hierarchical regressions were used to examine associations among violent victimization and perpetration and suicide attempts among adolescents who reported suicide ideation. The first step of the model consisted of demographic covariates (age, gender, race, and parents' income). The second step of the model consisted of depressive symptoms, non-violent delinquency, binge drinking, and marijuana use. The third step of the model consisted of violent victimization and perpetration. The fourth step of the model consisted of the interaction between violent victimization and perpetration. Given that suicide attempts were assessed on an ordinal scale with unequal intervals, analyses were estimated in M*plus* version 7 using WLSMV, which has demonstrated favorable properties over other estimation methods when specifying asymmetric ordinal outcomes (Li, 2014). Variables were centered prior to creating interaction terms. Full information maximum likelihood (FIML) missing data analysis was used to estimate low levels of missing data (ranging from 1% to 5%, although income was missing 13.2%). The magnitude and direction of all effects were similar with and without FIML estimation.

Results

Preliminary analyses

Descriptive statistics and bivariate correlations for all study variables are displayed in Tables 1 and 2, respectively. A total of n = 433 (52.7%) experienced some form of

Table 1. Descriptive statistics for key study variables.

	Range	M	SD
Binge Drinking	1–7	2.01	1.48
Marijuana Use	1–120	3.35	11.03
Non-violent Delinquency	0–3	0.45	0.47
Depressive Symptoms	0–3	0.93	0.50
Violence Perpetration	0–3	0.27	0.51
Victimization	0–2	0.25	0.35
Suicide Attempts		N	%
0 times	–	587	71.8
1 time	–	131	16.0
2 or 3 times	–	64	7.8
4 or 5 times	–	10	1.2
6 or more times	–	25	3.1

Notes: Study N = 821.

Table 2. Bivariate correlations among study variables.

	2	3	4	5	6	7	8	9	10	11	12	13
1. Age	−.10*	−.03	−.01	−.01	−.02	.18*	.14*	.00	.12*	−.03	−.04	−.04
2. Gender		.06	.03	−.05	.02	−.09*	−.16*	−.18*	.13*	−.23*	−.25*	.03
3. Black			−.02	−.08*	−.07	−.16*	−.02	−.11*	.01	.04	.04	.06
4. Hispanic				−.01	−.04	.03	.03	.01	.03	.06	.08	.03
5. Other					.01	−.01	−.06	.00	.04	−.03	−.01	.00
6. Income						.03	.02	−.04	−.12*	−.03	−.07	−.09*
7. Binge Drinking							.37*	.40*	.15*	.23*	.24*	.11*
8. Marijuana Use								.32*	.18*	.26*	.21*	.07
9. Non-violent Delinquency									.15*	.50*	.43*	.22*
10. Depressive Symptoms										.11*	.12*	.14*
11. Violence Perpetration											.61*	.26*
12. Victimization												.22*
13. Suicide Attempts												

Notes: *p < .05. Gender coded 1 = Male, 2 = Female.

victimization in the past year and n = 253 (30.8%) experienced some form of perpetration in the past year. Approximately 28% of youth who reported suicide ideation attempted suicide at least once in the past year, with 12.1% attempting suicide multiple times in the past year. In general, lower income, greater binge drinking, greater engagement in non-violent delinquency, greater depressive symptoms, greater experiences with violent victimization, and greater experiences with violence perpetration were correlated with higher suicide attempts (Table 2).

Victimization, perpetration, and suicide attempts

A stepwise hierarchical regression was used to examine associations between violent victimization and perpetration and suicide attempts among youth who endorsed past-year suicide ideation. The standardized estimates, unstandardized estimates, and standard errors from this model are displayed in Table 3. Demographic characteristics were entered into the first step of the

Table 3. Standardized estimates, unstandardized estimates, and standard errors for hierarchical multiple regression predicting suicide attempts.

	Suicide Attempts among Ideators															
	Step 1				Step 2				Step 3				Step 4			
	β	B	SE	p	β	B	SE	p	β	B	SE	p	β	B	SE	p
Age	-.06	-.04	.03	.21	-.08	-.05	.03	.08	-.07	-.04	.03	.15	-.07	-.04	.03	.16
Gender	.06	.13	.09	.15	.09*	.20	.10	.05	.13*	.28	.11	.01	.12*	.26	.11	.02
Black	.08*	.22	.11	.05	.11*	.29	.12	.01	.09*	.25	.12	.04	.10*	.26	.12	.03
Hispanic	.04	.16	.20	.44	.03	.13	.20	.52	.01	.06	.20	.78	.02	.08	.20	.71
Other	.02	.10	.21	.64	.02	.08	.21	.70	.02	.09	.22	.70	.02	.08	.22	.72
Income	-.16*	.01	.01	.03	-.12	.01	.01	.07	-.10	.01	.01	.15	-.10	.01	.01	.12
Binge Drinking					-.08	-.05	.03	.09	-.07	-.05	.03	.13	-.07	-.05	.03	.13
Marijuana Use					.01	.01	.01	.94	-.01	.01	.01	.77	-.02	.00	.01	.64
Non-violent Delinquency					.20*	.21	.05	.01	.13*	.14	.05	.01	.12*	.13	.06	.02
Depression					.12*	.01	.01	.01	.11*	.01	.01	.01	.11*	.01	.01	.01
Violence Perpetration									.03	.04	.07	.59	-.01	-.01	.08	.95
Violence Victimization									.13*	.14	.06	.03	.08	.09	.06	.18
Perpetration x Victimization													.11*	.06	.03	.04
R^2		.04				.10				.13				.14		
ΔR^2						.06*				.03*				.01		

Notes: *$p < .05$. Gender coded 1 = Male, 2 = Female. The overall model statistics were χ^2 (13) = 7.36, CFI = 1.00, RMSEA = < 0.01.

model. Income and race differences were the only significant effects in the first step of the model, with greater income associated with lower suicide attempts and Black youth experiencing a higher number of suicide attempts relative to non-Black youth among adolescents who reported suicide ideation. Overall, demographic characteristics explained 4% of the variance in suicide attempts. Binge drinking, marijuana use, non-violent delinquency, and depressive symptoms were entered into the second step of the model. Greater endorsement of non-violent delinquency and depressive symptoms were associated with a higher number of suicide attempts among adolescents who reported suicide ideation. Overall, binge drinking, marijuana use, non-violent delinquency, and depressive symptoms accounted for an additional 6% of variance in suicide attempts over demographic characteristics.

Violent victimization and perpetration were entered into the third step of the model. After accounting for demographic characteristics, binge drinking, marijuana use, non-violent delinquency, and depressive symptoms, we found that more frequent victimization experiences were associated with greater suicide attempts among adolescents who reported suicide ideation. Overall, these constructs explained an additional 3% of the variance in suicide attempts. The fourth and final step of the model consisted of a violence perpetration by violent victimization interaction. This interaction was significant and simple slope analyses were used to probe the nature of this interaction (Figure 1). These analyses indicate that violence perpetration was more strongly associated with suicide attempts for youth who experienced greater victimization ($\beta = .11$, $B = .134$, $SE = .054$, $p = .13$) relative to those who experienced less victimization ($\beta = .056$, $B = .124$, $SE = .151$, $p = .41$).

Discussion

Ideation-to-action frameworks for suicide behavior suggest that separate processes contribute to suicide ideation versus suicide attempts, which may help explain the

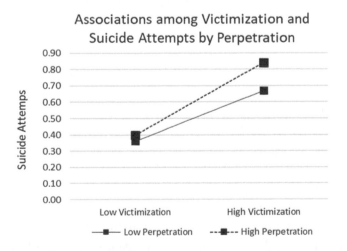

Figure 1. Interactive effect of victimization and perpetration on adolescents' suicide attempts.

discrepant rates of those who contemplate suicide and those who attempt suicide (Klonsky & May, 2015; O'Connor, 2011; Van Orden et al., 2010). While differences exist across theories, ideation-to-action frameworks highlight the role of the acquired capability for suicide in the process towards engaging in suicide behavior. Specifically, the IPTS describes how painful or provocative experiences drive increases in pain tolerance and fearlessness of death, which contribute to the acquired capability for suicide (Van Orden et al., 2010).

This study examined the associations between violent victimization and perpetration and suicide attempts in the past 12 months among youth who have reported past-year suicide ideation. Consistent with our main hypothesis, results indicated that violent victimization was associated with suicide attempts, even when accounting for demographic characteristics, depressive symptoms, and other externalizing behaviors that have been linked with suicide attempts in previous research (e.g., substance use and non-violent delinquency; May & Victor, 2018). Findings also indicated that the interaction of violence perpetration by victimization was associated with suicide attempts, demonstrating that the combination of victimization and perpetration has the strongest association with suicide attempts among adolescents who reported suicide ideation. Additionally, simple slopes analysis indicated that high levels of only victimization or perpetration were not significantly associated with suicide attempts.

One possible explanation of the current findings is that violent victimization and perpetration contribute to different elements of the acquired capability, as proposed by the IPTS (Van Orden et al., 2010). It may be that violent victimization is associated with an increase in pain tolerance, whereas violence perpetration is associated with decreased fear of death (and thus, increased willingness to engage in self-directed violent acts). The IPTS proposes that exposure to painful and provocative experiences results in increased pain tolerance via habituation to pain (Van Orden et al., 2010). Thus, repeated violent victimization, or violent victimization followed by a traumatic stress response (i.e., re-experiencing, intrusive cognitions, avoidance, and/or numbing), may serve to habituate adolescents to pain, increasing their acquired capability and accounting for the association between victimization and suicide attempts (Bryan & Anestis, 2011; Kaplow, Gipson, Horwitz, Burch, & King, 2014; Zuromski, Davis, Witte, Weathers, & Blevins, 2014).

Similarly, violent perpetration, including injuring or threatening others, involves exposure to physical danger and risk. Repeated experiences of perpetration may result in decreased fear of death in the face of physical danger – signaling an increase in the acquired capability for suicide. Thus, both violent victimization and perpetration may increase different aspects of the acquired capability for suicide, via mechanisms proposed by the IPTS.

Further, we may speculate that if violent victimization and perpetration differentially activate elements of the acquired capability, the joint presence of both violent victimization and perpetration may signal a heightened level of acquired capability, as would be predicted by the IPTS. Thus, individuals high in violent victimization but low in violence perpetration may have increased pain tolerance but may not have developed the fearlessness about death necessary to engage in self-directed violence. This would imply that either aspect of the acquired capability (pain tolerance or fearlessness about death) in isolation is not sufficient to result in suicide attempts. Additional research is needed to examine whether victimization and perpetration are differentially associated with pain tolerance or fearlessness about death. Future research should also attempt to replicate the interaction effect reported above.

In addition to the observed association between violent victimization and suicide attempts, non-violent delinquency remained significantly associated with suicide attempts in the final step of our model. While these behaviors do not expose people to pain as directly as experiences of violence, risky behaviors (e.g., drug sales, illegal activities, unprotected sex) may increase the acquired capability for suicide via gradual exposure to a lower grade of painful and provocative experiences or risk-taking more generally. Further, these behaviors may occur with greater frequency than violence exposure, providing greater opportunities for habituation to pain and/or fear of death. Future research should evaluate associations between non-violent delinquency and elements of the acquired capability for suicide.

Findings from this study have important implications for developmental conceptualizations of suicide risk. The association between violent victimization, perpetration, and suicide attempts may help explain age-related changes in suicide attempts across adolescence. Prior research has indicated that experiences of violent victimization, perpetration, and non-violent delinquency all increase during adolescence (Finkelhor et al., 2009; Moffitt, 1993), and evidence indicates an increase in suicide rates by age (Centers for Disease Control and Prevention (CDC), 2018a). Findings from this study suggest that risk for suicide may increase throughout adolescence due, in part, to increased exposure to painful and provocative experiences such as violent victimization, perpetration, and non-violent delinquency.

Implications for practice

Identifying specific painful or provocative experiences associated with suicide behavior may help us better understand the development of the acquired capability for suicide. Violent experiences directly expose people to pain and to the fear of death, providing opportunities for the acquired capability to develop. These findings also highlight the importance of regular assessment for trauma history (victimization) and violent and non-violent externalizing behaviors (perpetration and delinquency) in clinical practice. They suggest that histories of violent victimization, perpetration, or non-violent delinquency may be helpful in assessing suicide risk among youth. Specifically, when a client indicates thoughts of suicide, these factors may be of particular importance and may help clinicians make critical decisions regarding the safety of their client. The presence of a history of violent victimization and perpetration may indicate that an adolescent has an increased capability for suicide in the presence of suicide ideation. In addition, providers and professionals working in agencies that serve clients with heightened rates of violent victimization, perpetration, or non-violent delinquency (i.e., juvenile justice system, trauma-focused clinics, and agencies serving neighborhoods with high rates of community violence) should receive suicide risk assessment training and be aware of potentially heightened rates of suicide behavior among the populations they serve.

With regard to preventive interventions, ideation-to-action frameworks highlight key targets for suicide prevention when the acquired capability is present: The IPTS stresses reduction of suicide ideation as critical for those with the acquired capability (Joiner, 2005). The IMV and 3ST models also highlight the need to address other factors associated with suicide behavior, such as reducing access to lethal means, particularly when the acquired capability may be present. Practitioners working with adolescents exposed to violent victimization or perpetration should pay particular attention to lethal means restriction and providing services to address suicide ideation (e.g., the Collaborative Assessment and Management of Suicide; Jobes, 2012; the Safety Planning Intervention; Stanley & Brown, 2012).

Limitations and future directions

The findings of this study should be interpreted in the context of the strengths and weakness of the study design. Strengths include: (a) the use of a large national sample, (b) the large number of youth reporting recent suicide behavior, (c) examination of suicide attempts among those reporting suicide ideation, and (d) the use of an ideation-to-action framework. However, this study is limited by the use of cross-sectional data, which prevents examination of the directionality of the findings and causal interpretations, and by a limited number of mental health related variables, preventing an examination of the larger context around the transition from suicide ideation to suicide attempts. Future research should utilize a prospective, longitudinal study design to better evaluate the effects of violent victimization and perpetration experiences on suicide attempts across time. Additionally, the study relied on adolescent self-report and may have been subject to reporting biases. However, previous research has demonstrated that youth and parents frequently disagree when reporting on suicide related behaviors, so multiple informants may be of limited utility (Klaus, Mobilio, & King, 2009). Additional research is needed to more closely examine the associations between suicide-related behaviors and violence victimization and perpetration, as well as specific violent experiences that may contribute to suicide risk. Future studies should also evaluate whether violence victimization and perpetration are associated with hypothesized mechanisms of the acquired capability for suicide, namely fearlessness about death and increased pain tolerance. For example, examination of adolescent exposure to violence in relation to self-report measures of fearlessness about death (Ribeiro et al., 2014) or behavioral measures of pain tolerance (e.g., cold pressor or pressure algometer tasks; Pennings & Anestis, 2013) may help identify mechanisms by which violence victimization and perpetration are associated with suicide-related behaviors.

Conclusion

The current study examined the relations between violent victimization and perpetration and suicide attempts among a national sample of youth reporting suicide ideation. Violent victimization and the interaction between violent victimization and perpetration were associated with greater frequency of suicide attempts, even after accounting for demographic characteristics, depressive symptoms, and other non-violent externalizing behaviors. Non-violent delinquency was also significantly associated with suicide attempts in the final step of our model. These findings suggest that these experiences and behaviors may be important factors in the progression from suicide ideation to suicide attempts. Additionally, our findings suggest clinicians working with populations with high rates of violent victimization and perpetration should be aware of the potentially higher risk for suicide behavior amid the population they serve. Future research should examine the associations between these factors and mechanisms of ideation-to-action frameworks for suicide behavior, such as fearlessness of death, increased pain tolerance, and the subsequent acquired capability for suicide.

Disclosure statement

No potential conflict of interest was reported by the authors.

Funding

Support for this work was provided, in part, by a grant from the Substance Abuse and Mental Health Services Administration (SM-062111), given to Dr. Kaplow. This research uses data from Add Health, a program project directed by Kathleen Mullan Harris and designed by J. Richard Udry, Peter S. Bearman, and Kathleen Mullan Harris at the University of North Carolina at Chapel Hill, and funded by grant P01-HD31921 from the Eunice Kennedy Shriver National Institute of Child Health and Human Development, with cooperative funding from 23 other federal agencies and foundations. Special acknowledgment is due Ronald R. Rindfuss and Barbara Entwisle for assistance in the original design. Information on how to obtain the Add Health data files is available on the Add Health website (http://www.cpc.unc.edu/addhealth). No direct support was received from grant P01-HD31921 for this analysis,

ORCID

Evan E. Rooney ⓘ http://orcid.org/0000-0001-9773-1253

References

Anestis, M. D., Khazem, L. R., Mohn, R. S., & Green, B. A. (2015). Testing the main hypotheses of the interpersonal–Psychological theory of suicidal behavior in a large diverse sample of United States military personnel. *Comprehensive Psychiatry, 60*, 78–85. doi:10.1016/j.comppsych.2015.03.006

Arango, A., Opperman, K. J., Gipson, P. Y., & King, C. A. (2016). Suicidal ideation and suicide attempts among youth who report bully victimization, bully perpetration and/or low social connectedness. *Journal of Adolescence, 51*, 19–29. doi:10.1016/j.adolescence.2016.05.003

Borges, G., Nock, M. K., Medina-Mora, M. E., Hwang, I., & Kessler, R. C. (2010). Psychiatric disorders, comorbidity, and suicidality in Mexico. *Journal of Affective Disorders, 124*(1), 98–107. doi:10.1016/j.jad.2009.10.022

Bryan, C., & Anestis, M. (2011). Reexperiencing symptoms and the interpersonal-psychological theory of suicidal behavior among deployed service members evaluated for traumatic brain injury. *Journal of Clinical Psychology, 67*(9), 856–865. doi:10.1002/jclp.20808

Castellví, P., Miranda-Mendizábal, A., Parés-Badell, O., Almenara, J., Alonso, I., Blasco, M. J., … Piqueras, J. A. (2017). Exposure to violence, a risk for suicide in youths and young adults. A meta-analysis of longitudinal studies. *Acta Psychiatrica Scandinavica, 135*(3), 195–211. doi:10.1111/acps.12679

Centers for Disease Control and Prevention (CDC). (2018a). *Web-based injury statistics query and reporting system.* Retrieved from https://www.cdc.gov/injury/wisqars/index.html.

Centers for Disease Control and Prevention (CDC). (2018b). *1995–2017 Middle school youth risk behavior survey data.* Retrieved from http://nccd.cdc.gov/youthonline/

Czyz, E. K., Berona, J., & King, C. A. (2015). A prospective examination of the interpersonal-psychological theory of suicidal behavior among psychiatric adolescent inpatients. *Suicide & Life-Threatening Behavior, 45*(2), 243–259. doi:10.1111/sltb.12125

Deeds, B. G., Lagrange, R., Simoni-Wastila, L., & Peralta, L. (2007). 3: Understanding trends in youth violence: The role of gender, violent victimization and depression. *Journal of Adolescent Health, 40*(2), S15–S16. doi:10.1016/j.jadohealth.2006.11.046

DeVylder, J. E., Oh, H. Y., Nam, B., Sharpe, T. L., Lehmann, M., & Link, B. G. (2017). Prevalence, demographic variation and psychological correlates of exposure to police victimisation in four US cities. *Epidemiology and Psychiatric Sciences, 26*(5), 466–477. doi:10.1017/S2045796016000810

Dhingra, K., Boduszek, D., & O'Connor, R. C. (2015). Differentiating suicide attempters from suicide ideators using the integrated motivational–Volitional model of suicidal behaviour. *Journal of Affective Disorders, 186*, 211–218. doi:10.1016/j.jad.2015.07.007

Dhingra, K., Boduszek, D., & O'Connor, R. C. (2016). A structural test of the integrated motivational-volitional model of suicidal behaviour. *Psychiatry Research, 239*, 169–178. doi:10.1016/j.psychres.2016.03.023

Dhingra, K., Klonsky, E. D., & Tapola, V. (2018). An empirical test of the three-step theory of suicide in U.K. university students. *Suicide & Life-Threatening Behavior.* doi:10.1111/sltb.12437

Fergusson, D. M., Beautrais, A. L., & Horwood, L. J. (2003). Vulnerability and resiliency to suicidal behaviours in young people. *Psychological Medicine, 33*(1), 61–73.

Finkelhor, D., Turner, H., Ormrod, R., & Hamby, S. L. (2009). Violence, abuse, and crime exposure in a national sample of children and youth. *Pediatrics, 124*(5), 1411–1423. doi:10.1542/peds.2009-0467

Hann, D., Winter, K., & Jacobsen, P. (1999). Measurement of depressive symptoms in cancer patients. Evaluation of the Center for Epidemiological Studies Depression Scale (CES-D). *Journal of Psychosomatic Research, 46*, 437–443.

Harris, K. M., C. T. Halpern, E.Whitsel, J. Hussey, J. Tabor, P. Entzel, and J. R. Udry. 2009. The National Longitudinal Study of Adolescent to Adult Health: Research Design [WWW document]. URL: http://www.cpc.unc.edu/projects/addhealth/design.

Hepburn, L., Azrael, D., Molnar, B., & Miller, M. (2012). Bullying and suicidal behaviors among urban high school youth. *The Journal of Adolescent Health : Official Publication of the Society for Adolescent Medicine, 51*(1), 93–95. doi:10.1016/j.jadohealth.2011.12.014

Hill, R. M., & Pettit, J. W. (2014). Perceived burdensomeness and suicide-related behaviors in clinical samples: Current evidence and future directions. *Journal of Clinical Psychology, 70* (7), 631–643. doi:10.1002/jclp.22071

Ilgen, M. A., Burnette, M. L., Conner, K. R., Czyz, E., Murray, R., & Chermack, S. (2010). The association between violence and lifetime suicidal thoughts and behaviors in individuals treated for substance use disorders. *Addictive Behaviors, 35*(2), 111–115. doi:10.1016/j.addbeh.2009.09.010

Jobes, D. A. (2012). The Collaborative Assessment and Management of Suicidality (CAMS): An evolving evidence-based clinical approach to suicidal risk. *Suicide & Life-Threatening Behavior, 42*(6), 640–653. doi:10.1111/j.1943-278X.2012.00119.x

Joiner, T. E. (2005). *Why people die by suicide.* Cambridge, MA: Harvard University Press.

Kann, L., McManus, T., Harris, W. A., Shanklin, S. L., Flint, K. H., Queen, B., … Ethier, K. A. (2018). Youth risk behavior surveillance - United States, 2017. *Morbidity and Mortality Weekly Report. Surveillance Summaries (Washington, D.C.:2002), 67*(8), 1–114. doi:10.15585/mmwr.ss6708a1

Kaplow, J. B., Gipson, P. Y., Horwitz, A. G., Burch, B. N., & King, C. A. (2014). Emotional suppression mediates the relationship between adverse life events and adolescent suicide: Implications for prevention. *Prevention Science, 15*(2), 177–185. doi:10.1007/s11121-013-0367-9

Kessler, R. C., Borges, G., & Walters, E. E. (1999). Prevalence of and risk factors for lifetime suicide attempts in the national comorbidity survey. *Archives of General Psychiatry, 56*(7), 617–626.

Kimmel, D. (2014). Effects of adolescent violent victimization on adult depression: Testing heterogeneity for men and women. *Society and Mental Health, 4*(3), 179–196. doi:10.1177/2156869314527295

Kiriakidis, S. P. (2008). Bullying and suicide attempts among adolescents kept in custody. *Crisis: the Journal of Crisis Intervention and Suicide Prevention, 29*(4), 216. doi:10.1027/0227-5910.29.4.216

Klaus, N. M., Mobilio, A., & King, C. A. (2009). Parent–Adolescent agreement concerning adolescents' suicidal thoughts and behaviors. *Journal of Clinical Child & Adolescent Psychology, 38*(2), 245–255. doi:10.1080/15374410802698412

Klomek, A. B., Kleinman, M., Altschuler, E., Marrocco, F., Amakawa, L., & Gould, M. S. (2013). Suicidal adolescents' experiences with bullying perpetration and victimization during high school as risk factors for later depression and suicidality. *The Journal of Adolescent Health : Official Publication of the Society for Adolescent Medicine, 53*(1), S37–S42. doi:10.1016/j.jadohealth.2012.12.008

Klomek, A. B., Marrocco, F., Kleinman, M., Schonfeld, I. S., & Gould, M. S. (2007). Bullying, depression, and suicidality in adolescents. *Journal of the American Academy of Child & Adolescent Psychiatry*, *46*(1), 40–49. doi:10.1097/01.chi.0000242237.84925.18

Klonsky, E. D., & May, A. M. (2015). The three-step theory (3ST): A new theory of suicide rooted in the "ideation-to-action" framework. *International Journal of Cognitive Therapy*, *8* (2), 114–129. doi:10.1521/ijct.2015.8.2.114

Li, C. H. (2014). *The performance of MLR, USLMV, and WLSMV estimation in structural regression models with ordinal variables* (Unpublished doctoral dissertation). Michigan State University, East Lansing, MI.

May, A. M., & Klonsky, E. D. (2016). What distinguishes suicide attempters from suicide ideators? A meta-analysis of potential factors. *Clinical Psychology: Science and Practice*, *23* (1), 5–20.

May, A. M., & Victor, S. E. (2018). From ideation to action: Recent advances in understanding suicide capability. *Current Opinion in Psychology*, *22*, 1–6. doi:10.1016/j.copsyc.2017.07.007

Moffitt, T. E. (1993). Adolescence-limited and life-course-persistent antisocial behavior: A developmental taxonomy. *Psychological Review*, *100*, 674–701.

Nock, M. K., Borges, G., Bromet, E. J., Alonso, J., Angermeyer, M., Beautrais, A., … Williams, D. (2008). Cross-national prevalence and risk factors for suicidal ideation, plans and attempts. *The British Journal of Psychiatry*, *192*(2), 98–105. doi:10.1192/bjp.bp.107.040113

O'Connor, R. C. (2011). The integrated motivational-volitional model of suicidal behavior. *Crisis: the Journal of Crisis Intervention and Suicide Prevention*, *32*(6), 295–298. doi:10.1027/0227-5910/a000120

Oosterhoff, B., Kaplow, J. B., & Layne, C. M. (2016). Trajectories of binge drinking differentially mediate associations between adolescent violence exposure and subsequent adjustment in young adulthood. *Translational Issues in Psychological Science*, *2*(4), 371–381. doi:10.1037/tps0000092

Pennings, S. M., & Anestis, M. D. (2013). Discomfort intolerance and the acquired capability for suicide. *Cognitive Therapy and Research*, *37*(6), 1269–1275. doi:10.1007/s10608-013-9548-x

Resnick, M., Bearman, P., Blum, R., Bauman, K., Harris, K., Jones, J., … Udry, J. (1997). Protecting adolescents from harm: Findings from the national longitudinal study on adolescent health. *Jama*, *278*(10), 823–832.

Ribeiro, J. D., Witte, T. K., Van Orden, K. A., Selby, E. A., Gordon, K. H., Bender, T. W., … Thomas, E. (2014). Fearlessness about death: The psychometric properties and construct validity of the revision to the acquired capability for suicide scale. *Psychological Assessment*, *26*(1), 115–126. doi:10.1037/a0034858

Stanley, B., & Brown, G. K. (2012). Safety Planning Intervention: A brief intervention to mitigate suicide risk. *Cognitive and Behavioral Practice*, *19*(2), 256–264. doi:10.1016/j.cbpra.2011.01.001

Stewart, S. M., Eaddy, M., Horton, S. E., Hughes, J., & Kennard, B. (2017). The validity of the interpersonal theory of suicide in adolescence: A review. *Journal of Clinical Child & Adolescent Psychology*, *46*(3), 437–449. doi:10.1080/15374416.2015.1020542

Ten Have, M., de Graaf, R., van Dorsselaer, S., Verdurmen, J., Van't Land, H., Vollebergh, W., & Beekman, A. (2009). Incidence and course of suicidal ideation and suicide attempts in the general population. *The Canadian Journal of Psychiatry*, *54*(12), 824–833. doi:10.1177/070674370905401205

Thomas, H. J., Connor, J. P., Lawrence, D. M., Hafekost, J. M., Zubrick, S. R., & Scott, J. G. (2017). Prevalence and correlates of bullying victimisation and perpetration in a nationally representative sample of Australian youth. *Australian & New Zealand Journal of Psychiatry, 51*(9), 909–920. doi:10.1177/0004867417707819

Van Dulmen, M., Mata, A., Claxton, S., Klipfel, K., Schinka, K., Swahn, M., & Bossarte, R. (2013). Longitudinal associations between violence and suicidality from adolescence into adulthood. *Suicide & Life-Threatening Behavior, 43*(5), 523–531. doi:10.1111/sltb.12036

Van Orden, K. A., Witte, T. K., Cukrowicz, K. C., Braithwaite, S. R., Selby, E. A., & Joiner, T. E. (2010). The interpersonal theory of suicide. *Psychological Review, 117*(2), 575–600. doi:10.1037/a0018697

Zuromski, K. L., Davis, M. T., Witte, T. K., Weathers, F., & Blevins, C. (2014). PTSD symptom clusters are differentially associated with components of the acquired capability for suicide. *Suicide & Life-Threatening Behavior, 44*(6), 682–697. doi:10.1111/sltb.12098

Establishing a research agenda for child and adolescent safety planning

Christopher W. Drapeau ⓘD

ABSTRACT

Safety planning has been shown to reduce suicide risk and days in inpatient care among adults, but few studies have investigated how safety planning influences suicide-related outcomes among at-risk children and adolescents. This lack of research presents several avenues of research for researchers to explore. Aiming to establish a research agenda for safety planning research among youth, this paper outlines three areas of need in the research literature: 1) Facilitators and barriers influencing the use of safety plans among youth; 2) Parental involvement and parent-professional collaboration; and 3) Novel methods for safety planning development, modification, and application.

Suicide has become more frequent in the United States (U.S.) over the past decade (Centers for Disease Control and Prevention [CDC], n.d.), with rates rising among 10–74 year olds between 1999 and 2014 (Curtin, Warner, & Hedegaard, 2016). Among youth aged 5–18 years, the suicide rate has risen every year since 2012 (CDC, n.d.), increasing by 14.3% from 2016 to 2017. Although suicide is the tenth leading cause of death in the U.S., it has been the second leading cause of death among 5–18 year olds since 2011 (CDC, n.d.) accounting for 12,820 deaths from 2011–2017. Psychosocial interventions aimed at reducing suicide risk have shown promising results among adults (Brown & Jager-Hyman, 2014) and adolescents (Calear et al., 2016), and the National Action Alliance for Suicide Prevention recently identified clinical interventions that could close common gaps in healthcare for persons at risk for suicide (National Action Alliance for Suicide Prevention, 2018). One intervention proposed as filling one of the identified gaps (i.e., "Not Acting Effectively for Safety") is safety planning, a brief intervention that can lessen the risk for a suicide attempt by identifying potential coping strategies and supportive personal and professional contacts that can be utilized during a suicidal crisis (Stanley & Brown, 2012; Stanley et al., 2009).

Description of safety planning

Stanley and Brown (2012) outline six specific steps for completing the safety planning intervention (see Table 1 for a summary). The first step entails identifying personal warning signs of an imminent suicidal crisis. Stanley and Brown (2012) argue that an effective method for avoiding suicidal crises is addressing the issues contributing to the crisis before the crisis emerges. Noting specific warning signs that typically precede a suicidal crisis is one way to help the patient notice when a crisis is impending; thus, providing a chance to act before the crisis fully emerges. The warning signs identified as part of this initial step can include "personal situations, thoughts, images, thinking styles, moods, or behaviors" (Stanley & Brown, 2012, p. 258).

The second step includes identifying internal coping strategies (Stanley & Brown, 2012). This step focuses on listing activities that can be completed independently and will distract the patient from the suicidal crisis. It is postulated that these activities or coping strategies (e.g., exercising, taking a walk, etc.) can enhance "self-efficacy and ... help ... create a sense that suicidal urges can be mastered" (Stanley & Brown, 2012, p. 259). As part of this step, it is important to assess the likelihood that the patient will use the

Table 1. The six steps of Stanley and Brown's (2012) safety planning intervention.

Steps	Focus of Step	Sample Questions to Ask
Step 1	Identifying personal warning signs of an imminent suicide-related crisis	*How will you know when the safety plan should be used?*
Step 2	Using internal coping strategies	*What can you do on your own if you become suicidal again, to help yourself not to act on your thoughts or urges?* *What activities could you do to help take your mind off your problems even if it is for a brief period of time?*
Step 3	Utilizing social distractors	*Who helps you feel good when you socialize with them?* *Who helps you take your mind off your problems at least for a little while? You don't have to tell them about your suicidal feelings.* *Where can you go where you'll have the opportunity to be around people in a safe environment?*
Step 4	Contacting trusted individuals who can help resolve the suicide-related crisis	*Among your family or friends, who do you think you could contact for help during a crisis?* *Who is supportive of you and who do you feel that you can talk with when you're under stress?*
Step 5	Contacting mental health professionals and/or agencies	*Who are the mental health professionals that we should identify to be on your safety plan?* *Are there other health care providers?*
Step 6	Making the immediate environment(s) safe (lethal means reduction)	*What means do you have access to and are likely to use to make a suicide attempt or to kill yourself?* *How can we go about developing a plan to limit your access to these means?*

Note. Sample questions directly quoted from Stanley and Brown (2008). Researchers and clinicians will need to consider adapting the questions to fit the child or adolescent's developmental level (e.g., the word "socialize" in "Who helps you feel good when you socialize with them?" could be replaced with "talk" or "spend time").

identified coping strategies, including their ease of use, and rank order the priority of the identified activities based on perceived effectiveness. Additionally, it is important to explore for potential implementation barriers (e.g., lack of follow-up by clinicians, low patient confidence in plan, etc.) and collaboratively identify ways to overcome them if identified (Stanley & Brown, 2008).

The third step includes the identification of social distractors and social support. As hopefully is clear by the stepwise format of this intervention, each step should be enacted by the patient if the previous step was ineffective at diminishing suicide-related thoughts. If the internal coping strategies from step two prove unhelpful, step three will guide patients toward accessing "key social settings and people in their natural social environment who may help take them outside themselves and distract them from their suicidal thoughts and urges" and increase the opportunity for greater feelings of connectedness (Stanley & Brown, 2008, p. 7, 2012). Options for step three could include trusted peers or adults or "settings were socializing occurs naturally … [though] patients should be encouraged to exclude environments in which alcohol or other substances may be present" (Stanley & Brown, 2012, p. 259). A few examples of settings that may be helpful include coffee shops, festivals, places of worship, sports events, and local or internet interest groups. Although this step partly emphasizes seeking social support, it is important to note that such support is sought only for distraction from the suicidal crisis and not for seeking help specifically for it. The latter is the focus of step four should step three fail to alleviate suicide-related thoughts.

The fourth step includes identifying people the patient can contact to help resolve a suicidal crisis. When carrying out this step, the patient explicitly informs those identified as part of this step that they (the patient) are experiencing a suicidal crisis and in need of help (Stanley & Brown, 2012). Planning during this step should include a collaborative discussion between the clinician and patient regarding any advantages and/or disadvantages of disclosing suicide-related thoughts and behaviors to those sought after for support. The likelihood of disclosing thoughts to the identified individuals should also be discussed along with any hesitations toward disclosing (i.e., would the individual respond helpfully or exacerbate suicide risk?). Listing someone the patient feels close to on the safety plan is also recommended, as is sharing the safety plan with this individual (Stanley & Brown, 2012). However, it should be noted that the safety plan is meant to be "helpful and supportive and not a source of additional stress or burden" (Stanley & Brown, 2008, p. 9). It is possible that the patient may not feel comfortable sharing the finalized safety plan with anyone. In such instances, it is important to remember that identifying someone who will have access to the finalized safety plan is not a requirement for this step (Stanley & Brown, 2008).

The fifth step focuses on identifying professionals and/or agencies who can contacted when the patient is in crisis and the previous steps have failed to resolve the crisis. This should include the contact information of current mental health providers that the patient is willing to contact and any relevant professionals available during non-business hours (e.g., 24-hour emergency treatment facilities and support services like the National Suicide Prevention Lifeline). The purpose of this step is to emphasize that "appropriate professional help is accessible in a crisis and, when necessary, indicates how these services may be obtained (Stanley & Brown, 2012, p. 260). As with previous steps, it is important to explore for potential barriers that may dissuade patients from contacting the identified professionals and collaboratively identify ways to overcome these barriers if any are identified (Stanley & Brown, 2012).

The final step focuses on identifying ways to make the patient's immediate environment safe through limiting access to potentially lethal suicide attempt methods (Stanley & Brown, 2008). It is anticipated that addressing means restriction after identifying coping strategies at earlier steps of this intervention will help the patient notice that there are options other than attempting suicide and such a realization may lead to a greater openness to discuss the restriction of preferred suicide attempt method(s) (Stanley & Brown, 2012). For lethal methods (e.g., firearm), it is recommended that the patient avoid contact with the item and have a trusted, responsible adult safely store the item for a designated period of time. The designated person and the specific time period for storing the item should be noted as part of this step. Additionally, clinicians should note the specific behaviors the patient will engage in to make their environment safe. Clinicians also should ask all patients if they have access to firearms regardless of whether firearms were noted as a potential suicide attempt method (Stanley & Brown, 2012).

Stanley and Brown (2012) emphasize that the safety planning intervention should be completed collaboratively and clinicians should assess the patient's reaction to the plan, and their likelihood of using it, following completion. If the patient seems ambivalent about using the safety plan, this presents an opportunity to identify existing barriers and collaboratively problem solve with the patient. It is important to note that although the safety planning intervention has been proposed as a standalone intervention (Erbacher & Singer, 2018), the intervention can complement suicide risk assessments and was originally developed for emergency or acute care settings (i.e., Emergency Departments, crisis hotlines, etc.; Stanley & Brown, 2012). However, the intervention can be (and has been) used in other settings, such as psychiatric inpatient settings, military and correctional settings, and school settings (Erbacher, Singer, & Poland, 2015; Stanley & Brown, 2012).

Research on safety planning

The need for brief, effective interventions for reducing suicide risk and improving treatment compliance is supported by studies showing poor compliance with treatment recommendations following discharge from inpatient treatment or emergency departments (Granboulan, Roudot-Thoraval, Lemerle, & Alvin, 2001; Litt, Cuskey, & Rudd, 1983; Monti, Cedereke, & Öjehagen, 2003; O'Brien, Holton, Hurren, Watt, & Hassanyeh, 1987; Piacentini et al., 1995; Spirito, Stanton, Donaldson, & Boergers, 2002). A number of safety planning tools have been created to address these concerns and the Joint Commission (2016) now recommends collaboratively developing a safety plan with all patients presenting with suicide ideation (and reviewing the developed safety plan during each subsequent meeting until patient suicide risk subsides).

Research among adults employing safety planning tools (i.e., crisis response planning) shows quicker resolution of suicide ideation, reductions in suicide attempts, and fewer days in inpatient treatment compared to patients who were given safety contracts (Bryan et al., 2017). For those unfamiliar with safety contracts, these can include 1) a written agreement between the patient and clinician that the patient will refrain from suicide-related behavior over a specific period of time, 2) a contingency plan in the event that a patient feels unable to honor their contract, and 3) any patient and clinician contract-related responsibilities (Rudd, Mandrusiak, & Joiner, 2006). These contracts have shown limited effectiveness (Edwards & Sachmann, 2010) and have been criticized (see Stanley & Brown, 2012) for focusing on what the patient will not do during a crisis (i.e., attempt suicide) instead of focusing on what they can do (which is the emphasis of the safety planning intervention).

Reductions in suicide-related thoughts and behaviors, and less days in inpatient treatment, have also been shown in more recent adult studies Bryan, May, et al., 2018; Bryan, Mintz, et al., 2018). Furthermore, a recent cohort-comparison study among adults aged 18 years and older showed that Stanley and Brown's (2012) Safety Planning Intervention, combined with a structured telephone follow-up contact, led to a reduction in suicide-related behavior and an increased likelihood of attending mental health treatment compared to those receiving care-as-usual following discharge from an emergency department (Stanley et al., 2018). Research also suggests that adult patients find safety planning helpful in reducing their risk for attempting suicide (Stanley et al., 2016) and emergency department staff members have found the intervention useful for increasing adult patient safety, adult patient connection with follow-up services, and staff confidence in safely discharging adult patients (Chesin et al., 2017). However, it is notable that few published studies have examined the use of safety planning interventions with children and adolescents at risk for attempting suicide. Given this gap in the research literature, the current author is proposing a few critical areas for future research to address for the purpose of establishing a research agenda for child and adolescent safety planning.

Current youth research and gaps in the literature

The studies that have investigated safety planning among youth have shown promising results thus far. A randomized control trial of 36 hospitalized teens showed that a motivational interview (MI) -enhanced safety planning intervention (MI-SafeCope) led to greater self-reliance in coping with suicide-related thoughts and a higher likelihood of using the safety plan to manage thoughts of suicide (Czyz, King, & Biermann, 2018). In addition, a pilot study of a psychosocial intervention among 463 adolescent inpatients showed decreased odds of hospitalization and emergency room usage in the 12 months following inpatient discharge after completing intervention modules on safety plan development and enhancing life (Wolff et al., 2018). Furthermore, a qualitative study aimed at developing a safety plan phone application described positive perceptions regarding the usefulness of safety plans among adolescents with a history of suicide risk, their parents, and clinicians (Kennard et al., 2015).

Although the results from the aforementioned studies are encouraging, more research is needed in order to determine the replicability and generalizability of results. The most pressing question to answer at present is whether safety planning interventions reduce youth suicide risk as effectively as they appear to reduce risk in adult samples and if this effectiveness generalizes to all youth (and across all settings in which the intervention is currently used with children and adolescents). The few studies published to this point give the impression of an affirmative answer to this question for inpatient adolescents; however, replications among adolescents and research among children are required before concluding definitively that safety planning decreases suicide risk among children and adolescents.

Additionally, it is unknown if significant differences exist between the safety plans that are utilized among youth versus those safety plans that are not utilized at all. At this point, we know very little about what influences the use and usefulness of safety plans among youth, including clinician, patient, and family factors that improve the utilization and effectiveness of safety planning interventions in keeping youth at-risk for attempting suicide safe. What follows are three areas proposed by the current author as a research agenda for expanding our understanding of safety planning among children and adolescents. Sample research questions for each of the subsequent areas are also provided (see Table 2).

Table 2. Sample research questions for child and adolescent safety planning intervention research.

General	*How does the safety planning intervention influence suicide risk in children and adolescents?*
	Are there differences in intervention fidelity among health and mental health professionals working across divergent settings (e.g., school, hospital, outpatient, emergency room, etc.)? What is the incidence of safety planning intervention training among the professional settings serving children and adolescents? How are professionals trained in the intervention in theses settings?
Area 1: Safety Plan Facilitators and Barriers	*Does a collaborative approach to safety planning reduce the incidence of psychiatric hospitalization for children and adolescents? How does developmental level (or cognitive ability) affect the completion and usage of the safety plan?*
	How does the safety planning intervention affect suicide risk in the school setting? Does the effectiveness of the intervention differ based on the setting in which it is developed?
	What is the relationship between lack of clinician follow up on the safety plan and safety plan usage among children and adolescents? How does clinician comfort with, and attitudes toward, safety planning influence safety plan usage among children and adolescents? Does greater comfort with, and more positive attitudes toward, safety planning from the clinician predict more positive attitudes toward safety planning in the child and/or adolescent?
Area 2: Parent-Professional Collaboration	*What is the relationship between parental involvement in safety planning interventions among children and adolescents and safety plan usage and/or effectiveness? Does parenting style moderate this relationship?*
	When is parental involvement in the safety planning process no longer helpful to the child or adolescent patient?
	What clinician behaviors do parents find helpful or harmful to involving them in the safety planning process?
	Are there differences in intervention fidelity between parents and clinicians trained in the safety planning intervention?
Area 3: Novel Applications of Safety Planning with Youth	*How do safety planning phone applications influence suicide risk in children and adolescents? How do safety planning phone applications compare to safety planning interventions delivered in-person?*
	Which safety planning phone applications are most effective in reducing youth suicide risk? Does the effectiveness of these apps differ based on developmental level (child versus adolescent)?
	What are the effects of a peer-led safety planning intervention delivered in-person, via texting, or via social media on child or adolescent suicide risk?
	What are child and adolescent client perceptions of the safety planning intervention? Does satisfaction with the intervention differ depending on whether the intervention is peer-led, clinician-led, or parent-led?

Note. Given concerns about how well youth interventions translate from research to practice or "real-world" settings (see Weisz, Krumholz, Santucci, Thomassin, & Ng, 2015), it is recommended that researchers consider the sample questions (and any research questions related to safety planning) with implementation and transportability in mind.

Safety plan facilitators and barriers

Safety planning research among military veterans suggests that safety plans are most meaningful and successful at reducing subsequent psychiatric hospitalizations when clinicians are competent and collaborative in completing safety plans with patients (Gamarra, Luciano, Gradus, & Stirman, 2015; Kayman, Goldstein, Dixon, & Goodman, 2015; Levandowski, Cass, Miller, Kemp, & Conner, 2017). Additional facilitators of safety plan use include discussion of the safety plan during outpatient sessions, recounting helpful advice from clinicians when discussing the safety plan intervention in past sessions, and the patient being able to share their safety plan with supportive contacts (Kayman et al., 2015). Although some of these facilitators may be observed among youth, there likely will be some divergence due to environmental and developmental differences between military veterans and youth. For instance, children and adolescents may spend most of their time in a school setting compared to veterans who could be employed across an array of occupational specialties and living more independently than youth. Thus, the settings in which safety planning interventions are employed may differ between these populations (e.g., youth receiving the intervention in a school setting and veterans receiving the intervention in a Veterans Health Administration hospital or medical center).

Although research has been conducted among military veterans, there remains a paucity of research exploring for facilitators among children in general and outside of inpatient settings for adolescents. The frequency and quality of mental health professional safety plan training across the settings that youth may receive the intervention is also unknown. The absence of such research provides a starting point for those interested in identifying facilitators for youth and for those wishing to explore whether facilitators vary depending on developmental level or environment (e.g., school, hospital, outpatient, etc.).

Barriers likely will also differ between adults and youth for similar reasons, but a few barriers reported among a small sample of adults may have relevance for youth. These include lack of follow-up on safety plan usage by clinicians, the patient not keeping track of their safety plan, and the coping skills and contacts noted on the plan being less useful than expected (Gamarra et al., 2015). Additional patient-specific barriers to consider include a perceived lack of privacy (i.e., difficulty concealing the safety plan from others), a mismatch between identified coping activities and the patient's preferred coping style, patient doubts about using the plan when feeling depressed, patient perception that the burden of carrying out the plan will rest entirely on them, and a lack of access to professional care after hours and on weekends (Kayman et al., 2015).

For teens, one qualitative study of inpatient adolescents, parents, and clinicians revealed a belief among both parents and clinicians that adolescent emotional dysregulation acted as a barrier to using safety plans during times of distress (Kennard et al., 2015). Other barriers identified from this study (for inpatient adolescents) included low motivation, poor accessibility of the safety plan, and a desire not to include others (Kennard et al., 2015). An additional adaptation to consider when thinking of facilitators and barriers is the inclusion of minor peers on the safety plan as persons who could help during a crisis (B. Stanley, personal communication, September 30, 2018).

Research has also examined whether an electronic reminder to complete a safety plan when suicide-related ideation, a suicide attempt plan, or a nonfatal suicide attempt are noted in the patient note could improve the incidence of safety planning among clinicians serving outpatient adolescents at-risk for attempting suicide (Reyes-Portillo et al., 2018). Although results showed that adolescents reporting suicide risk who saw clinicians receiving the electronic health record alerts were three times more likely to complete a safety plan with the clinician compared to the control group, only 50.7% of these adolescents completed a safety plan (Reyes-Portillo et al., 2018). The researchers postulated that the timing of the alert likely affected the study outcomes since the alert could only occur when the clinician was document-ing the session, a practice that typically occurs after a patient leaves. However, future research could investigate whether such electronic alerts are helpful for clinicians and their patients when alerts occur in real time. Additionally, research examining clinician comfort with, and attitudes toward, safety planning may be useful given that clinicians who felt more comfortable with safety planning reported greater satisfaction with the safety planning alert (Reyes-Portillo et al., 2018). As with the facilitator research, there remains no research (to the author's knowledge) that has explored for barriers to safety plan usage among children.

Parent-professional collaboration

Family and parent-focused involvement in youth treatment appears to have a positive influence on parenting practices and patient outcomes (Carr, 2014; West, Sanders, Cleghorn, & Davies, 2010), with some evidence suggesting that changes in parenting practices serve as an important mechanism in youth behavioral change (Forehand, Lafko, Parent, & Burt, 2014). However, it is unknown if parenting practices might serve as a barrier or facilitator to safety plan usage among youth. Furthermore, research has yet to explore for family and/or peer factors that may influence safety plan usage, such as whether a peer group with multiple or high-status peers (e.g., Kiesner, Cadinu, Poulin, & Bucci, 2002) utilizing a safety planning intervention (or a suicide prevention phone application with a safety planning component) increases utilization.

To this point, one study has shown that a safety planning intervention enhanced with motivational interviewing can motivate parents to encourage safety plan usage (Czyz et al., 2018). However, the results of a qualitative study suggest that a large number of parents have little to no involvement in the safety planning development process and know very little about the content in the safety plan as a result (Kennard et al., 2015). In addition, the majority of parents in the study were unaware of the location of their child's safety plan, but believed that the plan was generally helpful. Almost all of the adolescents in the study reported that some parental involvement would be helpful in safety plan development (Kennard et al., 2015).

Future research is needed in order to better understand why some parents are not integrated in the safety planning process and how to best integrate their involvement. Additional research could examine whether barriers to parental involvement exist among the differing milieus in which safety plans are developed for youth (e.g., emergency departments, schools, outpatient clinics, etc.) and how clinician factors can facilitate or impede parental involvement. Another possible avenue of research includes piloting a safety planning parent or family education intervention focused on increasing parent/family member empowerment related to identifying suicide risk and helping with safety plan implementation (similar to family-led programs from organizations like the National Alliance on Mental Illness [see review by Hoagwood et al., 2010] or parent education interventions that have been developed for parents of children with Autism [see Brookman-Frazee, 2004]).

Novel applications of safety planning with youth

A study of 76 child and adolescent inpatients showed that 66% of the youth discharged from the unit owned a smartphone and the majority of the sample reported interest in downloading a suicide prevention phone application following their discharge (Gregory, Sukhera, & Taylor-Gates, 2017). These results suggest that smartphone applications may be a promising tool for safety planning development and implementation, especially since smartphones may provide an alternative to aforementioned implementation barriers such as lack of privacy (Kayman et al., 2015) and poor accessibility (Kennard et al., 2015).

A systematic review in 2016 revealed that over 120 phone applications that refer to suicide exist, with about 14 of the 120-plus applications focusing on safety planning (Larsen, Nicholas, & Christensen, 2016). The researchers noted that the applications generally included only one suicide prevention strategy, but none of the reviewed applications were rigorously examined for effectiveness. The researchers noted that "With no regulation in the app marketplace, it currently falls on clinicians and consumers to delineate app quality" (Larsen et al., 2016, p. 11), but added that safety planning applications appear the "most comprehensive and evidence-informed" (p. 2). The latter conclusion is supported by a pilot study showing that an Australian safety planning smartphone application (BeyondNow) was related to increased coping with suicide risk and decreased severity and intensity of suicide-related thoughts when the application was used as an adjunct to mental health treatment (Melvin et al., 2018).

Given the potential interest in downloading suicide prevention phone apps following inpatient discharge among youth (Gregory et al., 2017), there remains an opportunity to explore novel applications of the safety planning intervention. Numerous apps have been developed thus far (Larsen et al., 2016), but more rigorous research is required in order to understand if these apps can reduce youth suicide risk (and how they compare to in-person safety planning). Additional novel applications to consider include a web-based safety planning intervention that could be self-guided or include peer support (see Possemato et al., 2018). In addition, training peers to deliver the safety planning intervention in-person and/or via other technological mediums (e.g., cell phone texting, social media via the internet, etc.) may be another application worthy of consideration. The web-based intervention application idea could also be extended to children, with the exception that guardians, family members, and/or a trusted adult could provide support rather than peers.

Conclusion

Safety planning is considered an essential component of a comprehensive approach to treating suicide risk, but its application is understudied among children and adolescents at risk for attempting suicide. Several avenues of research exist that can help us better understand if and how safety planning can be effective at preventing youth suicide. Specific areas of research emphasis include examining the facilitators and barriers influencing the quality and implementation of safety planning, parental involvement and parent-professional collaboration, and novel methods for safety planning development, modification, and implementation. With the rate of suicide rising in the US among most age groups (CDC, n.d.), and an increasing incidence of child and adolescent inpatient hospitalization related to suicide risk (Plemmons et al., 2018), identifying brief interventions that can reduce suicide attempt risk and also reduce the need for inpatient hospitalization seem needed. Safety planning appears to do both among adults (Bryan et al., 2018; Bryan et al., 2018, Bryan et al., 2017; Stanley et al., 2018) and now is the time to investigate if the intervention can do the same for at-risk youth.

Implications for practice

Safety planning is considered a best practice intervention for youth at risk for attempting suicide (Erbacher & Singer, 2018) even though the effectiveness of the intervention has not been rigorously examined among children and adolescents. The intervention currently appears effective for inpatient adolescents and has been used across multiple settings (e.g., hospital, outpatient, school, etc.). The ease of using the safety planning intervention across settings may increase opportunities for collaboration across professional disciplines. For instance, a child or adolescent's parent, physician, counselor, and school psychologist could obtain access to the finalized safety plan (assuming the appropriate permissions are granted) and be able to monitor the effectiveness of the safety plan in each of the environments in which they observe the patient and collaboratively adapt the plan with the patient if necessary. As outlined earlier in this paper, adult research has shown that safety planning can reduce the frequency of suicide attempts and days spent in inpatient treatment. If similar findings are observed among children and adolescents, this intervention should be paired with suicide risk assessments and could provide a promising alternative to psychiatric hospitalization.

To clarify, the current author is not suggesting that safety plans be abandoned until more evidence supporting their use is obtained. Completing a comprehensive safety plan has been recommended as a suggested general practice when suicide risk is formulated as being "high" by the clinician (see Baerger, 2001). Since legal courts "expect clinicians to take reasonable steps to prevent suicide" (Obegi, 2017, p. 456), an argument can be made that completing a safety planning intervention with a child or adolescent thinking of attempting suicide is an attempt to do just that. Thus, it is recommended that this practice continue, but with the understanding that more research is needed.

It is anticipated that adapting the intervention for preadolescent children may be needed given differences in cognitive ability, and level of independence, compared to adolescents. For instance, children may not understand the concept of a lethal method or the permanency of death and may require greater parental involvement to access resources needed to contact supports noted in the safety plan. Readers are encouraged to review the assessment guidelines provided by Ridge Anderson, Keyes, and Jobes (2016) to generate ideas for approaching safety planning with younger children. For instance, it may be helpful to have the child draw pictures of personal warning signs to ensure that the precipitators of their suicidal crises are fully understood (rather than relying solely on verbal report).

Acknowledgments

The author would like to thank Dr. Barbara Stanley for reviewing and providing feedback on the initial draft of this manuscript.

Disclosure statement

No potential conflict of interest was reported by the author.

ORCID

Christopher W. Drapeau ⓘ http://orcid.org/0000-0002-1304-5369

References

Baerger, D. R. (2001). Risk management with the suicidal patient: Lessons from case law. *Professional Psychology: Research and Practice, 32*, 359–366. doi:10.1037//0735-7028.32.4.359

Brookman-Frazee, L. (2004). Using parent/clinician partnerships in parent education programs for children with autism. *Journal of Positive Behavior Interventions, 6*, 195–213. doi:10.1177/10983007040060040201

Brown, G. K., & Jager-Hyman, S. (2014). Evidence-based psychotherapies for suicide prevention: Future directions. *American Journal of Preventive Medicine, 47*, S186–S194. doi:10.1016/j.amepre.2014.06.008

Bryan, C. J., May, A. M., Rozek, D. C., Williams, S. R., Clemans, T. A., Mintz, J., & Burch, T. S. (2018). Use of crisis management interventions among suicidal patients: Results of a randomized controlled trial. *Depression & Anxiety, 35*, 619–628. doi:10.1002/da.22753

Bryan, C. J., Mintz, J., Clemans, T. A., Burch, T. S., Leeson, B., Williams, S., & Rudd, M. D. (2018). Effect of crisis response planning on patient mood and clinician decision making: A clinical trial with suicidal U.S. soldiers. *Psychiatric Services, 69*, 108–111. doi:10.1176/appi.ps.201700157

Bryan, C. J., Mintz, J., Clemans, T. A., Leeson, B., Burch, T. S., Williams, S. R., … Rudd, M. D. (2017). Effect of crisis response planning vs. contracts for safety on suicide risk in U.S. Army Soldiers: A randomized clinical trial. *Journal of Affective Disorders, 212*, 64–72. doi:10.1016/j.jad.2017.01.028

Calear, A. L., Christensen, H., Freeman, A., Fenton, K., Grant, J. B., van Spijker, B., & Donker, T. (2016). A systematic review of psychosocial suicide prevention interventions for youth. *European Child & Adolescent Psychiatry, 25*, 467–482. doi:10.1007/s00787-015-0783-4

Carr, A. (2014). The evidence base for family therapy and systemic interventions for child-focused problems. *Journal of Family Therapy, 36*, 107–157. doi:10.1111/1467-6427.12032

Centers for Disease Control and Prevention, National Center for Health Statistics. (n.d.). *CDC wide-ranging online data for epidemiologic research (WONDER) online database.* Retrieved from https://wonder.cdc.gov/

Chesin, M. S., Stanley, B., Haigh, E. A. P., Chaudhury, S. R., Pontoski, K., Knox, K. L., & Brown, G. K. (2017). Staff views of an emergency department intervention using safety planning and structured follow-up with suicidal veterans. *Archives of Suicide Research, 21*, 127–137. doi:10.1080/13811118.2016.1164642

Commission, T. J. (2016). *Sentinel event alert 56: Detecting and treating suicide ideation in all settings.* Retrieved from https://www.jointcommission.org/assets/1/18/SEA_56_Suicide.pdf

Curtin, S. C., Warner, M., & Hedegaard, H. (2016). *Increase in suicide in the United States, 1999-2014. NCHS data brief, no 241.* Hyattsville, MD: National Center for Health Statistics.

Czyz, E. K., King, C. A., & Biermann, B. J. (2018). Motivational interviewing-enhanced safety planning for adolescents at high suicide risk: A pilot randomized controlled trial. *Journal of Clinical Child and Adolescent Psychology.* Advance online publication. doi:10.1080/15374416.2018.1496442

Edwards, S. J., & Sachmann, M. D. (2010). No-suicide contracts, no-suicide agreements, and no-suicide assurances: A study of their nature, utilization, perceived effectiveness, and potential to cause harm. *Crisis, 31*, 290–302. doi:10.1027/0227-5910/a000048

Erbacher, T. A., & Singer, J. B. (2018). Suicide risk monitoring: The missing piece in suicide risk assessment. *Contemporary School Psychology, 22*, 186–194. doi:10.1007/s40688-017-0164-8

Erbacher, T. A., Singer, J. B., & Poland, S. (2015). *Suicide in schools: A practitioner's guide to multi-level prevention, assessment, intervention, and postvention.* New York, NY: Routledge.

Forehand, R., Lafko, N., Parent, J., & Burt, K. B. (2014). Is parenting the mediator of change in behavioral parent training for externalizing problems of youth? *Clinical Psychology Review, 34*, 608–619. doi:10.1016/j.cpr.2014.10.001

Gamarra, J. M., Luciano, M. T., Gradus, J. L., & Stirman, S. W. (2015). Assessing variability and implementation fidelity of suicide prevention safety planning in a regional VA healthcare system. *Crisis, 36*, 433–439. doi:10.1027/0227-5910/a000345

Granboulan, V., Roudot-Thoraval, F., Lemerle, S., & Alvin, P. (2001). Predictive factors of post-discharge follow-up care among adolescent suicide attempters. *Acta Psychiatrica Scandinavica, 104*, 31–36. doi:10.1034/j.1600-0447.2001.00297.x

Gregory, J. M., Sukhera, J., & Taylor-Gates, M. (2017). Integrating smartphone technology at the time of discharge from a child and adolescent inpatient psychiatry unit. *Journal of the Canadian Academy of Child and Adolescent Psychiatry, 26*, 45–50. Retrieved from https://www.ncbi.nlm.nih.gov/pmc/articles/PMC5349282/

Hoagwood, K. E., Cavaleri, M. A., Olin, S. S., Burns, B. J., Slaton, E., Gruttadaro, D., & Hughes, R. (2010). Family support in children's mental health: A review and synthesis. *Clinical Child and Family Psychology Review, 13*, 1–45. doi:10.1007/s10567-009-0060-5

Kayman, D. J., Goldstein, M. F., Dixon, L., & Goodman, M. (2015). Perspectives of suicidal veterans on safety planning: Findings from a pilot study. *Crisis, 36*, 371–383. doi:10.1027/0227-5910/a000348

Kennard, B. D., Biernesser, C., Wolfe, K. L., Foxwell, A. A., Craddock Lee, S. J., Rial, K. V., ... Brent, D. A. (2015). Developing a brief suicide prevention intervention and mobile phone application: A qualitative report. *Journal of Technology in Human Services, 33*, 345–357. doi:10.1080/15228835.2015.1106384

Kiesner, J., Cadinu, M., Poulin, F., & Bucci, M. (2002). Group identification in early adolescence: Its relation with peer adjustment and its moderator effect on peer influence. *Child Development, 73*, 196–208. doi:10.1111/1467-8624.00400

Larsen, M. E., Nicholas, J., & Christensen, H. (2016). A systematic assessment of smartphone tools for suicide prevention. *Plos ONE, 11*(4), 1–14. doi:10.1371/journal.pone.0152285

Levandowski, B. A., Cass, C. M., Miller, S. N., Kemp, J. E., & Conner, K. R. (2017). An intervention with meaning: Perceptions of safety planning among veteran health administration providers. *Crisis, 38*, 376–383. doi:10.1027/0227-5910/a000433

Litt, I. F., Cuskey, W. R., & Rudd, S. (1983). Emergency room evaluation of the adolescent who attempts suicide: Compliance with follow-up. *The Journal of Adolescent Health, 4*, 106–108. doi:10.1016/S0197-0070(83)80028-X

Melvin, G. A., Gresham, D., Beaton, S., Coles, J., Tonge, B. J., Gordon, M. S., & Stanley, B. (2018). Evaluating the feasibility and effectiveness of an Australian safety planning smartphone application: A pilot study within a tertiary mental health service. *Suicide and Life-Threatening Behavior.* Advance online publication. doi:10.1111/sltb.12490

Monti, K. M., Cedereke, M., & Öjehagen, A. (2003). Treatment attendance and suicidal behavior 1 month and 3 months after a suicide attempt: A comparison between two samples. *Archives of Suicide Research, 7*, 167–174. doi:10.1080/13811110301581

National Action Alliance for Suicide Prevention: Transforming Health Systems Initiative Work Group. (2018). *Recommended standard care for people with suicide risk: Making health care suicide safe.* Washington, DC: Education Development Center, Inc.

O'Brien, G., Holton, A. R., Hurren, K., Watt, L., & Hassanyeh, F. (1987). Deliberate self-harm and predictors of outpatient attendance. *The British Journal of Psychiatry, 150,* 246–247. doi:10.1192/bjp.150.2.246

Obegi, J. H. (2017). Probable standards of care for suicide risk assessment. *Journal of the American Academy of Psychiatry and the Law, 45,* 452–459. Retrieved from http://jaapl.org/

Piacentini, J. M., Rotheram-Borus, M. J., Gillis, J. R., Graae, F., Trautman, P., Cantwell, C., ... Shaffer, D. (1995). Demographic predictors of treatment attendance among adolescent suicide attempters. *Journal of Consulting and Clinical Psychology, 63,* 469–473. doi:10.1037/0022-006X.63.3.469

Plemmons, G., Hall, M., Doupnik, S., Gay, J., Brown, C., Browning, W., ... Williams, D. (2018). Hospitalization for suicide ideation or attempt: 2008-2015. *Pediatrics, 141,* 6. doi:10.1542/peds.2017-2426

Possemato, K., Johnson, E. M., Emery, J. B., Wade, M., Acosta, M. C., Marsch, L. A., ... Maisto, S. A. (2018). A pilot study comparing peer supported web-based CBT to self-managed web CBT for primary care veterans with PTSD and hazardous alcohol use. *Psychiatric Rehabilitation Journal.* Advance online publication. doi:10.1037/prj0000334

Reyes-Portillo, J. A., Chin, E. M., Toso-Salman, J., Blake Turner, J., Vawdrey, D., & Mufson, L. (2018). Using electronic health record alerts to increase safety planning with youth at-risk for suicide: A non-randomized trial. *Child & Youth Care Forum, 47,* 391–402. doi:10.1007/s10566-018-9435-4

Ridge Anderson, A., Keyes, G. M., & Jobes, D. A. (2016). Understanding and treating suicidal risk in young children. *Practice Innovations, 1,* 3–19. doi:10.1037/pri0000018

Rudd, M. D., Mandrusiak, M., & Joiner, T. E. (2006). The case against no-suicide contracts: The commitment to treatment statement as a practice alternative. *Journal of Clinical Psychology, 62,* 243–251. doi:10.1002/jclp.20227

Spirito, A., Stanton, C., Donaldson, D., & Boergers, J. (2002). Treatment-as-usual for adolescent suicide attempters: Implications for the choice of comparison groups in psychotherapy research. *Journal of Clinical Child and Adolescent Psychology, 31,* 41–47. doi:10.1207/S15374424JCCP3101_06

Stanley, B., Brown, G., Brent, D., Wells, K., Poling, K., Curry, J., ... Hughes, J. (2009). Cognitive behavior therapy for suicide prevention (CBT-SP): Treatment model, feasibility and acceptability. *Journal of the American Academy of Child and Adolescent Psychiatry, 48,* 1005–1013. doi:10.1097/CHI.0b013e3181b5dbfe

Stanley, B., & Brown, G. K. (2008). *Safety plan treatment manual to reduce suicide risk: Veteran version.* Retrieved from https://www.mentalhealth.va.gov/docs/VA_Safety_planning_manual.pdf

Stanley, B., & Brown, G. K. (2012). Safety planning intervention: A brief intervention to mitigate suicide risk. *Cognitive and Behavioral Practice, 19,* 256–264. doi:10.1016/j.cbpra.2011.01.001

Stanley, B., Brown, G. K., Brenner, L. A., Galfalvy, H. C., Currier, G. W., Knox, K. L., ... Green, K. L. (2018). Comparison of the safety planning intervention with follow-up vs. usual care of suicidal patients in the emergency department. *JAMA Psychiatry, 75,* 894–900. doi:10.1001/jamapsychiatry.2018.1776

Stanley, B., Chaudhury, S. R., Chesin, M., Pontoski, K., Bush, A. M., Knox, K. L., & Brown, G. K. (2016). An emergency department intervention and follow-up to reduce suicide risk in the VA: Acceptability and effectiveness. *Psychiatric Services, 67,* 680–683. doi:10.1176/appi.ps.201500082

Weisz, J. R., Krumholz, L. S., Santucci, L., Thomassin, K., & Ng, M. Y. (2015). Shrinking the gap between research and practice: Tailoring and testing youth psychotherapies in clinical care contexts. *Annual Review of Clinical Psychology, 11,* 139–163. doi:10.1146/annurev-clinpsy-032814-112820

West, F., Sanders, M. R., Cleghorn, G. J., & Davies, P. S. W. (2010). Randomised clinical trial of a family-based lifestyle intervention for childhood obesity involving parents as the exclusive agents of change. *Behaviour Research and Therapy, 48,* 1170–1179. doi:10.1016/j.brat.2010.08.008

Wolff, J. C., Frazier, E. A., Weatherall, S. L., Thompson, A. D., Liu, R. T., & Hunt, J. I. (2018). Piloting of COPES: An empirically informed psychosocial intervention on an adolescent psychiatric inpatient unit. *Journal of Child & Adolescent Psychopharmacology, 28,* 409–414. doi:10.1089/cap.2017.0135

The potential use of CAMS for suicidal youth: building on epidemiology and clinical interventions

David A. Jobes, Genesis A. Vergara, Elizabeth C. Lanzillo, and Abby Ridge-Anderson

ABSTRACT

It is vital to better understand and effectively treat suicide, as it remains a leading cause of death for youth. The present article discusses the epidemiology of suicidal outcomes for youth and provides an overview of existing treatments. The "Collaborative Assessment and Management of Suicidality" (CAMS) – an evidence-based suicide-specific treatment – is presented, followed by a discussion of the potential benefits of adapting it to youth. Patient-defined "suicidal drivers," which are identified and targeted within CAMS-guided treatment, may be especially pertinent to suicidal youth who are in the beginning stages of grappling with their experience related to suicide. Current efforts to adapt CAMS for suicidal adolescents and children are described. Crucially, with further development and rigorous clinical research, adaptations of CAMS may one day provide an empirically-proven and reliable approach to reducing suicide risk in adolescents and children.

The notion of young people taking their own lives seems to run against our cultural and adult sensibilities. The topic is by its nature deeply uncomfortable to consider; the idea that a child as young as 4 could terminate his or her own life in an intentional manner may be astonishing, even unthinkable, to many. In this article we endeavor to tackle this difficult topic from an epidemiological perspective, followed by a review of effective clinical approaches based on the extant research literature. We will then explore the promise of adapting and applying to youth populations the "Collaborative Assessment and Management of Suicidality" (CAMS), an intervention that has proven to be effective with suicidal adults.

The epidemiology of youth suicide

As the second leading cause of death among youth ages 10–17 years (Centers for Disease Control and Prevention [CDC], 2016), suicide among young people is a major public health issue in the United States. Over the past 15 years, the age-adjusted youth suicide rates have risen by 24% (Curtin, Warner, & Hedegaard, 2016; Plemmons et al., 2018). While suicide is rarer prior to the onset of adolescence, it still ranks as the 9th leading cause of death for children aged 5–11 years (CDC, 2016). More common than completed suicide are suicidal thoughts and behaviors. Among adolescents aged 12–17 years, lifetime prevalence rates range between 19.8% and 24.0% for suicidal ideation and 3.1% and 8.8% for suicide attempts (Cha et al., 2018; Nock, Borges, et al., 2008). Notably, adolescents who experience suicidal thoughts are at greater risk of attempting suicide. Most adolescents who transition from ideation to attempt do so within 1–2 years of ideation onset (Glenn et al., 2017). This is marked by distinct clinical presentations (Nock et al., 2013).

While our understanding of youth suicide remains limited, various demographic patterns have been identified. Consistent with trends observed among adults, female adolescents are more likely to experience suicidal thoughts and attempts than their male counterparts, but male adolescents are more than twice as likely to die by suicide than females (Cha et al., 2018). However, this sex difference does not appear until approximately age 11 (Cha et al., 2018; Nock & Kazdin, 2002). Studies have also demonstrated age-related racial disparities in youth suicide, with the highest rate of suicide among indigenous youth (Centers for Disease Control and Prevention, 2016). Though findings among other racial groups are nuanced, recent data have revealed a significant age-related racial disparity among black and white youth, in which the suicide rate among youth younger than 13 years is approximately two times higher for black children compared to white children (Bridge et al., 2018). A similar trend was found in a study that examined deaths by suicide in children (aged 5–11 years) and early adolescents (aged 12–14 years); black children made up 36.8% of deaths by suicide in the 5–11 year old sample as compared to 11.6% in the early adolescent sample (Sheftall et al., 2016). Potential explanations for this racial disparity include disproportionate exposure to violence or traumatic stressors among black youth and increased challenges to accessing mental health services for black youth compared with non-black youth (Sheftall et al., 2016). There is a strong need for additional research aimed at confirming and expanding these explanations and further elucidating the underlying mechanisms driving this racial disparity.

An elevated prevalence of suicidal thoughts and behaviors has also been observed among lesbian, gay, bisexual, transgender and questioning (LGBTQ) youth compared to their heterosexual counterparts (Cha et al., 2018). Importantly, the impact of sexual minority status appears to be influenced by degree and availability of social support. For example, LGB youth living in an "unsupportive county" (defined by low proportion of: same-sex couples, registered Democrats, gay-straight alliances in schools, and school policies to protect LGB students) had a 20% higher risk of attempting suicide than their LGB peers living in more supportive communities (Cha et al., 2018; Hatzenbeulher, 2011). In addition to these demographic variables, several psychosocial correlates and risk factors associated with suicidal thoughts and behaviors have been identified. Among the environmental risk factors, childhood trauma, bullying, and academic pressure show consistent associations with increased suicidal risk.

Childhood trauma

Numerous studies have demonstrated that children who experience physical, sexual, or emotional abuse are at significantly higher risk for suicidal ideation, suicide attempts, and completed suicide (Cha et al., 2018; Joiner et al., 2007; Jokinen et al., 2010; Lanzillo, Horowitz, & Pao, 2018; Rajalin, Hirvikoski, & Jokinen, 2013). A study examining the effect of preadolescent physical abuse on adolescent suicidal behavior revealed a significant association between preadolescent abuse and elevated risk of suicidal ideation and attempt that was not mediated by contextual factors such as attachment to family or friends, internalizing or externalizing pathology, or life events (Lanzillo et al., 2018; Salzinger, Rosario, Feldman, & Ng-Mak, 2007). Another study examined suicide risk following childhood sexual abuse and found that the suicide rate was over ten times greater than the national rate among youth who experienced childhood sexual abuse (Lanzillo et al., 2018; Plunkett et al., 2001).

Bullying

There is extensive evidence highlighting the association between bullying and risk for suicide among youth. Findings suggest that for boys, being the perpetrator or the victim of bullying poses an increased risk for suicidal thoughts and behavior. Among girls, those who are victims of bullying are more likely to engage in suicidal behavior compared to girls who are neither perpetrators nor victims of bullying (Klomek et al., 2009; Lanzillo et al., 2018). A study examining risk for suicide in pediatric patients who presented to the emergency department found that over half (55%) of patients who reported recent bullying victimization screened positive for suicide risk (Lanzillo et al., 2018; Stanley, Horowitz, Bridge, Wharff, & Teach, 2016). As the use of social media and technology among youth continues to rapidly increase, recent research has focused on the effects of cyberbullying on suicidality. Findings indicate that cyberbullying has comparable, or potentially stronger effects, than traditional forms of bullying (Bauman, Toomey, & Walker, 2013; Cha et al., 2018; Hinduja & Patchin, 2010; Van Geel, Vedder, & Tanilon, 2014); however, more research is needed to further explore this relationship.

Academic pressure

The prevalence of "suicide clusters" in high schools known for their academic pressure reveals that such stress has the potential to trigger suicidal behavior (Lanzillo et al., 2018; Scelfo J., 2015). A suicide cluster exists when multiple deaths by suicide occur within an accelerated timeframe and/or in close geographical proximity (Gould, Wallenstein, & Davidson, 1989; Robertson, Skegg, Poore, Williams, & Taylor, 2012). For example, in 2009 the Palo Alto region of California witnessed the suicide deaths of five teens over the course of nine months. Approximately five years later, the region experienced another suicide cluster when four teens died by suicide (Rosin, 2015).

The causative factors leading to suicide clusters are complex and the subject of ongoing research. Conditions such as highly competitive and demanding academic environments may contribute to the occurrence of suicide clusters. Evidence also supports the theory that suicidal behavior can be "contagious" in that it can be modeled – directly or indirectly – from one individual to another (Gould & Lake, 2013). In response to suicide clusters, Joshi and colleagues (2015) suggest that death may be a more appealing escape to youth experiencing significant academic stress. Moreover, an individual's ability to develop alternatives to suicide may be inhibited in this context. Prevention efforts specific to school-based mental health education and promotion are warranted (Joshi et al., 2015). Much research addressing the relationship between academic stress and suicidal behavior has focused on East Asian populations (Lanzillo et al., 2018). Cultural factors may influence the way academic pressure manifests among youth; however, comparative research is warranted.

Psychopathology

Beyond environmental risk factors, a history of psychopathology is a well-established risk factor for suicidal thoughts and behavior. Cash and Bridge (2009) indicate that at least one psychiatric disorder is present in up to 80–90% of youth who attempt or die by suicide, with the most common diagnoses being mood, anxiety, conduct, and substance use disorders (Cash & Bridge, 2009; Lanzillo et al., 2018). Despite the established risk posed by the presence of psychiatric disorders, it is critical to not assume that only youth with mental illness are at heightened risk for suicide. In fact, a recent study examining antecedents of death by suicide among youth in England revealed that 61% of suicide decedents did not have a known psychiatric diagnosis (Lanzillo et al., 2018; Rodway et al., 2016). Conversely, the vast majority of youth with psychopathology will not develop suicidal thoughts or behavior. This highlights the challenges inherent to accurately predicting who will engage in suicidal behavior.

Biological factors

An emerging line of research explores the influence of biological processes on suicidality in youth. As the majority of studies on the biological underpinnings of suicidal behavior utilize cross-sectional designs, it is crucial to conceptualize these biological processes as *correlates* and not risk factors (Cha et al., 2018). Preliminary findings suggest that the hippocampus, involved in mood regulation and memory, and the dorsolateral prefrontal cortex, responsible for decision-making and emotional regulation, are structurally irregular in youth who have attempted suicide (Cha et al., 2018; Gosnell et al., 2016). These deficits can help to explain why and how individuals may choose to engage in suicidal behaviors. For example, poor decision-making and limited emotion regulation may contribute to making suicide a viable option in response to distress (Jollant et al., 2005). The default mode network (DMN) has also been found to be abnormally connected in adolescent attempters, suggesting that DMN irregularities may be a biomarker for suicide risk (Cha et al., 2018; Zhang et al., 2016). In addition to the DMN, abnormalities in the executive control network (ECN) and salience network (SN) have also been found among suicidal adolescents (Ordaz, Goyer, Ho, Singh, & Gotlib, 2018). These three networks (DMN, ECN, and SN) are involved in cognitive processes related to self-regulation and goal-directed behaviors (ECN), understanding of self and of one's place in the world (DMN), and interpretation of goal-relevant and threatening stimuli (SN) (Ordaz et al., 2018). As such, under- or over-activation of these networks in an adolescent's developing brain is likely to impair the adolescent's ability to effectively solve problems, regulate their emotions, manage and maintain satisfying interpersonal relationships, and have a sense of self-efficacy and ability to cope with stressors. In other words, disruptions in these networks are associated with many of the known risk factors for suicidal ideation and behaviors. Identification of abnormal network connectivity may improve our ability to understand, predict, and track suicide risk with the use of implicit and physiological measures. Research findings in this area are thus far limited by small samples and lack of replication, but neuroimaging research is a promising frontier.

Current approaches to preventing and treating youth suicidality

There is a paucity of research on interventions for suicidal teens and children particularly using randomized controlled trials (RCTs) which, along with RCT *replication* studies, are the definitive gold standard for determining what treatments are effective in a *causal* way (Cha et al., 2018; Glenn, Franklin, & Nock, 2015). Nonetheless, preliminary studies have been conducted on various psychotherapies. The reviews and meta-analyses that have been conducted on this target population all point to the need for more research on treatments for suicidal youth, particularly using longitudinal and RCT designs (Cha et al., 2018; Glenn et al., 2015; Ougrin, Tranah, Stahl, Moran, & Asarnow, 2015). Overall, the majority of psychotherapies for suicidal youth have been interpersonal, cognitive-behaviorally-oriented, and skills-based in their approaches, with a strong emphasis placed on parental and youth considerations.

Most of the research conducted on treatments for suicidal youth has been done with adolescent samples, although there have been some studies on children as young as 8– 11 years of age (Asarnow et al., 2011; Harrington et al., 1998; Huey et al., 2005; Perepletchikova et al., 2011). Treatments for suicidal youth have focused on the immediate reduction of suicidal outcomes (e.g., ideation, attempts). These interventions have primarily been studied for their ability to improve symptoms among those with a history of suicidal thoughts/behaviors. Efforts to decrease youth suicides also include a range of approaches and programs designed for youth with no history of suicidality, with the goal .of preventing suicidal thoughts and behaviors, rather than intervening after the fact.

Following a brief discussion of universal and targeted prevention efforts, the current review emphasizes interventions that have been adapted or developed for suicidal youth, with suicide-related outcomes as the primary target within RCT designs. Although many existing interventions for youth target psychiatric disorders that may include suicidality as a symptom (e.g., depression, borderline personality disorder), the present review centers on treatments that target suicide and related suicidal thought and behaviors as *primary* outcomes so that we may build on previous work that has increasingly called for a trans-diagnostic assessment of and treatment of suicide outcomes (Cha et al., 2018; Jobes, 2000; Nock et al., 2013).

Prevention

Prevention efforts are essential for reducing youth suicides, yet much more research is needed in this area. Prevention efforts for suicide can broadly take various forms: *universal* for everyone; *selective* for individuals that share a risk factor for suicide; and *indicated* for those with suicide risk but not receiving treatment for it (Cha et al., 2018; Katz et al., 2013; Robinson et al., 2013).

Universal

One universal prevention program is *Signs of Suicide* (SOS) – a school-wide, evidence-based prevention program for middle and high school youth. It consists of psychoeducation with a cognitive-behavioral element and screening for suicide and its risk factors (Gilman & Chard, 2015). Two studies found that it significantly lowered suicidal behavior in comparison to a control group, and improved adaptive attitudes and knowledge about suicide (Aseltine & DeMartino, 2004; Schilling, Lawless, Buchanan, & Aseltine, 2014). However, there was no difference in help seeking (for self and others) between the SOS and control groups. *Sources of Strength* (SoS) is another universal prevention program that has produced promising results in training peer leaders to assist in suicide outreach in school settings (Wyman et al., 2010).

Selective

The *Family Check-Up and Family Bereavement Intervention* (Connell, McKillop, & Dishion, 2016; Sandler, Tein, Wolchik, & Ayers, 2016) aims to prevent suicidal behaviors among at-risk youth by focusing on the developmental importance of the family and conflict within this system. This prevention program has shown to lead to long-term reductions in suicide-related outcomes; while promising, more longitudinal research is needed.

Indicated

Suicide hotlines have not been studied in youth and have produced mixed findings for adults (Cha et al., 2018). Community postventions following a suicide are similarly lacking empirical support. Studies examining the benefits of postvention efforts for adults and or children that may have been impacted by a suicide death will need to consider the unique ecological systems inherent to the impact of a single suicide on a community (Bronfenbrenner, 1977).

Psychotherapies

Attachment-based family therapy

Developed by Diamond, Reis, Diamond, Siqueland, and Isaacs (2002) "ABFT" reduces self-injurious thoughts and behaviors by improving family relationships, particularly the attachment relationship within the parent-child dyad. ABFT posits a ruptured attachment as the source of an adolescent's suicidality, and the repair of this relationship is achieved through a combination of weekly individual, parent, and family sessions over the course of 3 months. One RCT found a reduction in suicide ideation in comparison to an enhanced usual care (EUC) group in an adolescent sample, with improvements maintained at 6-month follow-up. This is particularly noteworthy given that this was found in a diverse sample from minority backgrounds (Diamond et al., 2010). Moreover, this built on similar RCT findings assessing ABFT in comparison to a waitlist control group, where rapid reduction of suicide ideation was observed at posttreatment (Diamond et al., 2002). While promising, it is important to note that the comparison groups in both studies had a low rate of treatment completion, which raises questions about the robustness of the findings. Additionally, suicide *behaviors* were not assessed in either study.

Integrated cognitive-behavioral therapy

Developed by Esposito-Smythers, Spirito, Kahler, Hunt, and Monti (2011), "I-CBT" challenges maladaptive cognitions, affective processes, and behaviors. I-CBT consists of individual and family therapy sessions and a parent training component delivered over 12 months. The treatment is designed to be intensive, with a 6-month course of active treatment, 3 months of biweekly continuation sessions, and 3 months of monthly maintenance sessions. Initially, what is now considered I-CBT only included individual CBT with the adolescent (Spirito, Esposito-Smythers, & Wolff, 2018) and findings showed no differences in outcomes between the experimental intervention and supportive therapy, as both treatments led to reductions in suicidal ideation and attempts (Donaldson, Spirito, & Esposito-Smythers, 2005). However, a small RCT (n = 40) with adolescents with a history of suicide attempts and substance use disorders revealed that while both I-CBT (modified to include parent-training and family therapy) and enhanced standard care (ESC) led to reductions in suicidal ideation, I-CBT had significantly lower rates of suicide attempts at 18-month follow-up (Esposito-Smythers et al., 2011). With a demonstrated ability to reduce suicidal behavior, I-CBT is clearly a promising approach, yet more research and replication needs to be done to address several limitations. Less than one-fifth of the families in ESC completed treatment, compared to nearly three-fourths of the I-CBT families; although the number of sessions attended was controlled for, this discrepancy in treatment engagement and completion does raise questions about the mechanisms of change in I-CBT. Additionally, I-CBT was adapted for and tested in a sample of suicidal adolescents with a co-morbid substance use diagnosis. As such, the positive treatment effects of I-CBT may not generalize to suicidal youth who are not also struggling with substance use.

Dialectical behavioral therapy for adolescents

"DBT-A" (Miller, Rathus, Linehan, Wetzler, & Leigh, 1997) is a developmental adaptation of DBT, an intensive treatment originally developed to treat adults with borderline personality disorder (BPD; Linehan, 1993), a diagnosis that is highly associated with suicide and self-harm. Through individual therapy, group-based skills-training, and between session phone-coaching by the therapist as needed, DBT targets maladaptive affective and interpersonal processes. In order to address the specific needs of adolescents, Miller et al. (1997) adapted DBT-A by shortening the length of treatment, incorporating parents in individual therapy as needed, and adding a skills training group specifically for parents. Results from one RCT found that DBT-A reduced suicidal ideation in comparison to the control condition over the course of the treatment, yet this reduction was not maintained at the one-year follow-up (Mehlum et al., 2016, 2014). One non-randomized controlled study comparing DBT-A to treatment as usual (TAU) found no significant difference in number of suicide attempts in each group; however they did find that adolescents in the DBT-A group had significantly fewer psychiatric hospitalizations than those in the TAU group (Rathus & Miller, 2002). DBT-A has subsequently been established as an evidence-based treatment for suicidal adolescents, with demonstrated reductions in suicidality found in two or more independent RCTs (McCauley et al., 2018).

Of note, Perepletchikova et al. (2011) tested an adaptation of DBT for younger children in a 6-week feasibility pilot study (n = 11); adaptions included a range of modifications, including larger text in handouts, second grade reading level, and child-friendly pictures and examples. Perepletchikova and colleagues noted that the modified intervention maintained fidelity to the original principles of DBT, including the DBT skills, and they found that comprehension was high among participants. They found that their participants had increased coping skills and reductions in depressive and internalizing symptoms and suicidal ideation from pre- to post-treatment. Given the limited treatments available for pre-adolescent children, further examination of this innovative treatment, with larger samples, is much needed.

Interpersonal psychotherapy for youth in school settings

Developed by Tang, Jou, Ko, Huang, and Yen (2009), "IPT-A-IN" is a developmentally-sensitive intervention for adolescents, addressing interpersonal stressors and processes implicated in suicide and depression (Liu & Miller, 2014; Vergara, Stewart, Cosby, Lincoln, & Auerbach, 2019). IPT-A-IN specifically targets interpersonal stressors such as conflict or grief in order to lower suicidality and depression symptoms (Tang et al., 2009). In a sample of depressed adolescents, Tang et al. (2009) found a significant reduction in suicidal ideation from pre- to post-treatment in comparison to TAU after 6 weeks. There was also a reduction in internalizing symptoms in the treatment group, although it was unclear whether this reduction mediated or moderated the suicide ideation findings. However, the researchers did not assess for suicide attempt behaviors so the impact of IPT-A-IN on such behavior is unknown. There were also no follow-up outcomes reported, suggesting there is a need to assess the longer-term impact of this treatment. Future replication RCT studies examining the benefits of this promising treatment should also be examined using more clinically diverse populations.

Emergency department and safety planning

Much research has been conducted on the *SAFETY program* (Asarnow, Berk, Hughes, & Anderson, 2015; Asarnow, Hughes, Babeva, & Sugar, 2017), a 12-week CBT-based program with a strong family component designed to increase treatment engagement and reduce suicidal behavior in suicidal adolescents following admission to an emergency department for a suicidal crisis. The SAFETY program is an expansion of the *Family Intervention for Suicide Prevention* (FISP, Asarnow et al., 2011). FISP is a brief intervention which consists of one family-based session in the emergency department focused on means restriction, safety planning, and establishing a plan for follow-up treatment; this session is followed by a check-in phone call post-discharge. While Asarnow et al. (2011) found an increase in treatment compliance in comparison to TAU, they did not find a reduction in suicide outcomes for FISP. However, a subsequent development study found that the expanded SAFETY program was associated with a reduction in suicidal behavior and internalizing symptoms (Asarnow et al., 2015). The effectiveness of the SAFETY program was further demonstrated in a recent RCT, with adolescents in the SAFETY program condition showing significant reductions in suicide attempts and emergency department visits as compared to youth in the control condition (Asarnow et al., 2017). Although additional research is needed, this suicide-specific, family-based intervention shows promise as an emergent evidence-based treatment option for suicidal youth.

Pharmacological treatments

No RCTs have been conducted assessing pharmacological interventions for suicide outcomes in youth (Ougrin et al., 2015). The *Treatment of Adolescent Suicide Attempters* (TASA; Brent et al., 2009) study, however, has suggested that medication in combination with psychotherapy may be especially relevant to study in this population. Specifically, Brent et al. (2009) conducted a study where suicidal adolescents received either CBT for suicide prevention (CBT-SP), medication only, or combined CBT-SP and medication over 6 months. There were no significant differences in suicidal ideation or attempts between the treatment conditions. This was an open trial, meaning participants were offered the option of selecting which treatment they wanted to receive; since most participants opted to receive the combined form of treatment, it is essential to further examine pharmacological treatments in this population.

Psychiatric hospitalization

Our review would be remiss if we did not discuss the common practice of inpatient hospitalization of suicidal youth. As discussed elsewhere by Jobes et al. (2017), this is a sensitive and contentious topic within the field of suicide prevention wherein some have argued that sub-sets of suicides are actually *caused* by the hospitalization experience (Large, Ryan, Walsh, Stein-Parbury, & Patfield, 2014). Recent work by Czyz, Berona, and King (2016) has in fact shown that re-hospitalization for a suicidal teenager significantly predicts a more severe course of suicidal ideation and can be a strong indicator for a future suicide attempt. Typical hospital stays are diagnostically-focused, rather than focused on addressing suicide as the primary treatment target (Jobes, 2016; Jobes et al., 2017; Jobes, Au, & Siegelman, 2015). The National Action Alliance for Suicide Prevention (2018) has recently released a document entitled: "Recommended Standard Care for People with Suicide Risk: Making Healthcare Suicide Safe". Incredibly, prior to this effort there were *no* accepted clinical guidelines or recommendations that might help address this urgent public health issue. This important document outlines the need for effective assessment of suicide risk, frank discussions with patients and family members about restricting access to lethal means in the home environment, the value of stabilization planning, the recommended use of the National Suicide Prevention Lifeline (1-800-273-TALK), and the evidence-based value of follow-up "caring contacts." Widespread implementation of these practice guidelines should serve to reduce the economic and psychological costs of psychiatric hospitalizations for suicidal youth.

CAMS adaptations for suicidal youth

Having thoroughly reviewed the incidence of child and adolescent suicide and related morbidity one might presume an expansive scientific research literature for clinically treating and saving our youth from this major public health challenge. Yet as we have also discussed, the nascent evidence base for effective treatments for suicidal youth requires increased and ongoing research efforts, especially for children under the age of 12 (Ridge-Anderson, Keyes, & Jobes, 2016). As we have further noted, there are concerns about existing "go-to" interventions such as prescribing medication (often off-label) and routine inpatient hospitalizations that are at best insufficiently suicide-focused, and may even be contraindicated in some cases. Given these grave considerations, youth-oriented suicide treatment researchers are increasingly determined to create and disseminate effective clinical responses to suicidality among children and adolescents.

CAMS as proven suicide-specific treatment

The Collaborative Assessment and Management of Suicidality (CAMS, Jobes, 2006, p. 2016), is a suicide-specific therapeutic framework that has been shown to be effective in eight non-randomized clinical trials in a wide range of settings and suicidal populations (see reviews by Jobes, 2012; Jobes, Gregorian, & Colborn, 2018). CAMS has also been proven effective in three randomized controlled trials (RCTs) demonstrating the *causal* effectiveness of CAMS with suicidal adults (Andreasson et al., 2016; Comtois et al., 2011; Huh et al., 2018; Jobes et al., 2017). Importantly, these rigorous RCTs of CAMS *replicate* positive findings in support of CAMS both within and between independent laboratories.

As a flexible suicide-specific clinical framework, CAMS can be used across settings, disciplines, and theoretical orientations (Jobes et al., 2018). Central to CAMS is the use of the *Suicide Status Form* (SSF), a patient-centered multi-method assessment, treatment planning, and tracking tool, that measures a range of clinical outcomes and can simultaneously function as a comprehensive medical record of each therapy session. Current efforts with colleagues at Microsoft are underway to create an "e-SSF" that will interface with electronic medical records (EMRs) used in most health facilities, with plans to study the use of the e-SSF in future RCT research.

The SSF assessment aspects of CAMS have been previously shown to function as a "therapeutic assessment" in one meta-analysis (Poston & Hanson, 2010) and there is evidence that successfully treated CAMS patients appreciate the process and experience of engaging with providers using the SSF (Schembari, Jobes, & Horgan, 2016). A signature feature of CAMS which may be central to its effectiveness is the emphasis of having the *patient* define their own "suicidal drivers" which are the problems that compel them to consider suicide. It follows that within "standard" use of CAMS, patient-defined suicidal drivers are systematically targeted and treated over the course of clinical care (Jobes, 2016). Taken together, the accumulated research to date demonstrates the following *replicated* clinical trial results with adult samples: CAMS quickly reduces suicidal ideation in 6–8 sessions, decreases overall symptom distress, increases hope while decreasing hopelessness, decreases depression, and decreases Emergency Department (ED) visits in sub-samples of suicidal patients. Patients rate CAMS as more satisfactory than standard care and CAMS is routinely associated with better treatment retention.

Given these positive clinical and research findings, many clinicians are eager to use CAMS with suicidal adolescents and children. To this end, two preliminary papers have been published about possible adaptations and recommendations for using CAMS with suicidal youth based on clinical experience and some early exploratory research (O'Connor, Brausch, Ridge-Anderson, & Jobes, 2014; Ridge-Anderson et al., 2016). Investigations into the use of CAMS with adolescents and children are now underway with results pending regarding feasibility, effectiveness, and possible needed adaptations. We feel there are promising early results supporting the value of applying CAMS to young people, with preliminary indications that adolescents treated with CAMS experience significant reductions in suicidality and depression symptoms (Ridge-Anderson, Jobes, & Lento, 2017). However, we cannot *presume* that CAMS will work equally well with suicidal youth as it does with adults. Moreover, it is essential to ensure that a newly developed treatment *never does harm*. Given the import of the topic and the intense clinical needs, several research teams are diligently working to adapt CAMS as needed to ensure that it works effectively with suicidal youth.

Having thoroughly considered a range of possible names for adapted versions of CAMS to be used with suicidal adolescents and children, we have decided on "CAMS-4Teens" and "CAMS-4Kids." Both adaptations have at their cores the four defining "pillars" of the CAMS philosophy across its many uses and adaptations (Jobes et al., 2018). As described by Jobes (2016), fundamental to CAMS philosophy are the following essential considerations: 1) Empathy, 2) Collaboration, 3) Honesty, and 4) Suicide-focus.

Developing cams-4teens

What follows herein is a brief review of work being done to date in our on-going efforts to develop a proven and effective use of CAMS for suicidal teenagers, children, and their families that also addresses many of the needs that clinicians and systems have related to this topic.

Psychometrics of the SSF for youth

The psychometric validity and reliability of the SSF has been well-established with adult samples (Conrad et al., 2009; Jobes, Jacoby, Cimbolic, & Hustead, 1997). But a very common source of skepticism about using the SSF with adolescents is that the language may not be developmentally appropriate. It has been suggested that a teenager could not comprehend and therefore not accurately rate the variables that make up the "SSF Core Assessment" (i.e., Psychological Pain, Stress, Agitation, Self-Hate, Hopelessness, and Overall Risk of Suicide – Jobes, 2016). For example, we have received feedback that the concept of "Psychological Pain" could not be understood by teens or explained by providers; we have thus been urged for years to develop an adolescent version of the SSF so that youth can understand and use the tool. However, careful clinical research to date on this topic contradicts this common assumption and should assuage this skeptical concern. The SSF Core Assessment of constructs has been successfully used as part of the standard screening assessment done for years at the Mayo Clinic within their routine psychiatric intake practice. Indeed, Romanowicz, O'Connor, Schak, Swintak, & Lineberry (2013) published a study of more than 1100 youth (ages 8–18 years old) and found that the SSF variables were understandable to their patients and served as a valuable baseline assessment; their SSF data were used effectively to aid in optimal treatment decision-making.

More recently, Amy Brausch's research team at Western Kentucky University (e.g., Powers et al., 2018) has actively pursued a rigorous psychometric study of the SSF with suicidal teenagers. Preliminary analyses of their data from a sample of 67 suicidal teens indicate that the SSF Core Assessment is psychometrically valid and reliable and helps differentiate suicidal risk. These researchers also have useful preliminary data from adolescent Implicit Association Test results (IAT, Nock & Banaji, 2007) that may provide further psychometric support for the SSF with adolescents in the future. Feedback from this on-going line of psychometric research has confirmed that adolescent participants feel quite strongly that the wording of the SSF does not need to be changed for them to understand what is being assessed. Moreover, central to CAMS as a treatment approach is the opportunity to create "teachable moments"; we find that while teenage patients in our studies are quite able to understand SSF constructs, exploring their understanding of these constructs helps teens cultivate an evolved language to better describe their suicidal experience. In sum, research to date on the use of the SSF with youth suggests that the SSF has good acceptability and the potential for strong psychometric properties.

The CAMS for youth working group continues to discuss and refine modifications to standard SSF *administration* guidelines in order to address developmental needs specific to children and adolescents. For example, many of the domains that child and adolescent clinicians generally include in a standard clinical assessment have important implications in the assessment of suicide risk: Sleep, social media use, and bullying experiences should be routinely monitored as part of the SSF assessment process within CAMS-4Teens and CAMS-4Kids. Establishing such developmentally-relevant guidelines is an important component of the CAMS research agenda, which is unfolding across several different clinical settings.

Seattle children's hospital

A major foothold in the development of CAMS 4-Teens is taking place at Seattle Children's Hospital where Molly Adrian (2017) and her colleagues have been adapting the use of CAMS for suicidal teenagers seen at their medical center. One project is an archival study that will compare a clinical sample of 62 suicidal adolescents receiving CAMS to a control group created using propensity score matching. A second project is an on-going feasibility study to further refine adaptations for youth and families to gather data to pursue grant funding to conduct a feasibility CAMS study and a small RCT with the ultimate goal of conducting well-powered – perhaps multi-site – RCTs of CAMS-4Teens.

The cleveland clinic

Other pioneers in the use of CAMS with adolescents are Tatiana Falcone and Jane Timmons-Mitchell at the Cleveland Clinic where they have been looking into the inpatient use of CAMS and the use of CAMS at discharge/disposition as a possible optimal discharge plan for certain suicidal inpatient teens (Pao et al., 2017). They are now pursuing grant funding for this line of research that may address a number of clinical challenges.

Georgia juvenile justice system

Given the increased risk of suicide and self-harm in forensic settings, there have been efforts to adapt the use of CAMS in juvenile justice facilities in the state of Georgia. Significant modifications are required to use an intervention like CAMS in a forensic setting. For example, an incarcerated youth cannot be allowed to fill out the SSF with a pen as there is the potential for it to be weaponized. Nevertheless, an adapted version of CAMS has been used in this system with some measure of clinical success (Cardeli, 2015). We are continuing to explore the prospect of further adaptations of CAMS in such correctional settings with the goal of one day conducting a randomized controlled trial examining the impact of CAMS on suicidal risk and non-suicidal self-injury (NSSI) among juvenile inmates.

CAMS in the context of school mental health (SMH) programs

Led by Kurt Michael, J.P. Jameson, and their team at Appalachian State University (Michael & Jameson, 2017), CAMS has been effectively integrated into several school districts in western North Carolina as part of university-school partnerships titled Assessment, Support, and Counseling (ASC) Centers (Albright et al., 2013). In early 2017, the ASC Centers scaled up regional capacity to utilize CAMS by training 50 local providers, the majority of which served children and adolescents in schools. The use of CAMS as part of the ASC Centers is now entering its third year of implementation and it has been found to be a feasible and effective intervention that is readily and flexibly integrated into existing school-related systems of care including the Multi-Tiered Systems of Support (MTSS) Model (Michael, Jameson, Filbin, Rosston, & Butts, 2017).

Family considerations and the role of parents

As we have discussed at length elsewhere, one of the biggest issues of using CAMS with teenagers is the proper involvement of parents (O'Connor et al., 2014). In clinical work with adolescents and children, parental involvement is both a legal obligation and critical for successful outcomes. However, the level and nature of parental involvement that leads to successful outcomes with suicidal youth within CAMS has not yet been empirically evaluated. Anecdotally, we have observed a broad spectrum of potential parental attitudes that may impact their capacity to be constructively involved in treatment. These generally range from: 1) parents who feel angry, blamed, and defensive, with behavior that may undermine rather than optimize care; 2) parents who have a mixed, neutral, or minimal level of interest in and impact on treatment; and 3) parents who are eager to be positively involved and can play an indispensable adjunctive role within successful care. Beyond these three broad characterizations, the familial aspects impacting suicidal youth have long been well known (Wagner, 1997) and are a major focus within our feasibility research. Our team is focused on the importance of the CAMS experience being empathic, collaborative, honest, and suicide-focused – the core philosophy of the CAMS approach (Jobes, 2016). As CAMS clinicians and researchers, we are also determined that adaptations maintain a patient-centered and drivers-oriented approach. With a focus on the developmental needs of children and adolescents (patient-centered), and the common risk factors for youth suicidality (drivers-oriented), this likely means that parent involvement will be emphasized in all cases, regardless of parent and family functioning at the start of treatment. Thus, as we work to develop and study youth adaptations for CAMS, our goal is to understand not *whether*, but rather *how* and *when* to involve parents and caregivers.

As a general matter, teens take pride in being expert on many topics; in our experience of using CAMS clinically with teens they appreciate being acknowledged as *the* expert on their own suicidal experience (which we explicitly embrace within CAMS-guided care). It is thus our general impression that suicidal teens take to CAMS quite well because it is so explicitly patient-centered. The adherent CAMS clinician follows the adolescent's lead; what the youth says matters most both in terms of assessment and the treatment of their self-defined suicidal drivers. Nevertheless, parents' perspectives must also be considered given their pivotal role in terms of risk assessment, lethal means safety, and further treatment. Assessing and managing parents' attitudes about their child's participation in a suicide-specific treatment can be difficult because parents often feel blamed or implicated. We are thus working on developing parent assessments that can be used to inform decisions about the types of support or resources parents might need to enable them to be optimally helpful to their child. We feel strongly that a child's SSF assessment data should be shared with parents in a joint meeting with the CAMS clinician and the child patient, to help the parents better understand the nature and seriousness of their child's suicidality. It is also crucial for the parents to review, understand, and retain a copy of their child's *CAMS Stabilization Plan* (CSP) because they are often key players in any discussion of lethal means safety within the household environment. They may also be able to help support the coping strategies that are listed on their child's CSP. In some cases, parents may be invited to participate in the development of the CSP, depending on the child's preferences and needs. Finally, it is imperative that parents be made aware of their child's self-defined suicidal drivers which will be the targets of treatment within CAMS-guided care. We also would support the use of an explicit *Crisis Support Plan* (Bryan, Stone, & Rudd, 2011) so that parents can have a treatment-oriented document that helps guide their support as an adjunct to the effective care of their child.

There are individual, developmental, and practical issues to consider in determining *how* the SSF and CSP are most effectively administered to youth and parents. Time constraints and the child's age and level of functioning may determine whether the CSP is developed with the parent and the teen present, or whether it is developed with the teen and then shared with the parent. Parent functioning and family dynamics must be considered when deciding whether to share the SSF with parents while the teen is present, or perhaps in a separate conversation. We are working to develop and evaluate guidelines that will ensure clinical flexibility while providing much-needed empirically-informed guidance. Respect for the *patient's* preferences must always remain at the forefront of clinical decision-making within CAMS.

Developing cams-4kids

In 2016, Ridge-Anderson et al. critiqued the limited attention the larger field of suicide prevention has placed on the problem of suicidal risk in children under the age of 12. For example, there is only one major book focused on the suicidal child within the published literature (Pfeffer, 1986). Interestingly, early research revealed that some medical examiners as a matter of medicolegal policy refuse to certify a suicide of a child under the age of 12, arguing that a child that young could not knowingly intend to terminate their life (Jobes, Berman, & Josselson, 1987). Nevertheless, Bridge et al. (2015) have shown more recently data that 657 children died by suicide between 1993 and 2012 – a death toll that amounts to about 33 children per year in the United States. While early on we discussed the epidemiology of youth suicide (which mostly focuses on teens), valid data on the number of young child suicide attempts and data on childhood suicidal ideation are elusive. But given the death toll, we might reasonably speculate that thousands of pre-adolescent children have suicidal thoughts. Although it may seem beyond our cultural grasp as adults, child suicides do indeed occur each year in the United States. When a child acts deliberately to cause his or her own death, dismissing the child's intentions by labeling such a death as accidental or undetermined ultimately serves to undermine efforts to prevent future similar tragedies. Although it may be difficult to accept, some young children do experience and act on thoughts of suicide when faced with intolerable pain.

To address this rare but nevertheless appalling concern, a nascent research effort is now underway with Jeff Bridge and his research team at Columbus Nationwide Hospital to develop a highly adapted version of CAMS for suicidal children under the age of 12, based on pioneering innovations and modifications of CAMS which are described in more depth elsewhere (Ridge-Anderson et al., 2016). Clearly a suicide-specific intervention for a 5-year-old girl must be highly modified, as someone that young can neither typically read nor comprehend the complexity of the SSF or ideas like a suicidal driver. The CAMS philosophy can be employed and the SSF can provide valuable clinical guidance, but the intervention must be significantly broken down and gently explained to a child in a way that they can understand and appreciate. CAMS-4Kids is thus fully consistent with the overall CAMS philosophy which guides the therapeutic process, and it still emphasizes the key elements of what we believe makes the treatment successful for other suicidal populations. Just as in CAMS with adults, CAMS-4Kids providers endeavor to enter the world of the patient to understand and see suicidality through the eyes of the patient (Jobes, 2016). However, rather than starting with side-by-side seating as in standard CAMS, we start CAMS-4Kids on the floor with lots of blocks, coloring books, toys, and sticker books readily available. Ideas like *psychological pain* and *self-hatred* are presented and explained in empathic, developmentally-appropriate, and caring terms. Assessment and treatment in CAMS-4Kids takes more time, and a CAMS-4Kids clinician must exert considerable patience despite any internal sense of urgency they may feel in response to their reasonable fear and discomfort when faced with the suicidality of a young child. Children may need to take breaks during the assessment process, given the weighty and complex feelings they are exploring. Discussing one's own suicidality in depth is difficult for many patients, adults and children alike; working with young children requires particular care and a keen attunement to the child's cognitive and emotional capacities. Nonetheless, our clinical experience to date suggests that young children can and do benefit from suicide-specific treatment, and parents can play a key life-saving role in this work when they are skillfully engaged.

In our early clinical pilot work, we have lost two children under the age of 12 to suicide; another child was murdered at the hands of her father. Clearly, not all children at risk are going to make it and the work is sometimes simply harrowing. But it is also true that dozens of the children we have seen have had excellent outcomes. We are learning much about what it takes to help prevent a suicide in a young child and how to work effectively with families of children at risk. Clearly, this is serious and perilous work, but it simply must be done. To this end, our research team is determined to craft and responsibly develop a CAMS-4Kids manual that can be rigorously tested through RCT research to demonstrate that young lives can be saved.

Implications for practice

As the second leading cause of death for youth, suicide is a major public health concern. The present article reviews the epidemiology of suicidal outcomes, revealing childhood trauma, bullying, and biological differences as factors that contribute to suicidal thoughts and behaviors among children and adolescents. There are several existing clinical interventions and prevention efforts that seek to reduce youth suicide. These interventions generally target emotion regulation difficulties, maladaptive behaviors, and interpersonal stressors, include a family component, and were primarily developed for adolescents. While much progress has been made, this review reveals the need for more effective treatments, especially for children under the age of 12. We highlighted a suicide-specific treatment, CAMS, that has proven effective in suicidal adults. With developmentally-driven adaptations and an emphasis on the core pillars of the CAMS model – empathy, collaboration, honesty, and suicide-focus – we believe that ongoing research, dissemination, and implementation of CAMS-4Teens and CAMS-4Kids will contribute significantly to the goal of preventing the loss of young lives due to suicide. Ultimately, we seek to support children, caregivers, clinicians, and stakeholders in ensuring that all youth have the opportunity and capacity to experience the many joys and challenges of living a full life that is worth living, with both purpose and meaning.

Disclosure statement

David A. Jobes would like to disclose the following potential conflicts: grant funding for clinical trial research from the Department of Defense, the American Foundation for Suicide Prevention, and the National Institute of Mental Health; book royalties from American Psychological Association Press and Guilford Press; co-owner of CAMS-care, LLC (a clinical training/consulting company).

References

Adrian, M. (2017). *Adaptive decision-making for adolescent psychotherapy targeting suicidality* (Unpublished grant proposal).

Albright, A., Michael, K. D., Massey, C. S., Sale, R., Kirk, A., & Egan, T. E. (2013). An evaluation of an interdisciplinary rural school mental health program in Appalachia. *Advances in School Mental Promotion, 6*, 189–202. doi:10.1080/1754730X.2013.808890

Andreasson, K., Krogh, J., Wenneberg, C., Jessen, H. K. L., Krakauer, K., Gluud, C., & Nordentoft, M. (2016). Effectiveness of dialectical behavior therapy versus collaborative assessment and management of suicidality treatment for reduction of self-harm in adults with borderline personality traits and disorder - A randomized observer-blinded clinical trial. *Depression and Anxiety, 33*, 520–530. doi:https://doi.org/10.1002/da.22472

Asarnow, J., Baraff, L., Berk, M., Grob, C., Devich-Navarro, M., Suddath, R., ... Tang, L. (2011). Effects of an emergency department mental health intervention for linking pediatric suicidal patients to follow-up mental health treatment: A randomized controlled trial. *Psychiatric Services, 62*, 1303–1309. doi:10.1176/ps.62.11.pss6211_1303

Asarnow, J. R., Berk, M., Hughes, J. L., & Anderson, N. L. (2015). The SAFETY Program: A treatment-development trial of a cognitive-behavioral family treatment for adolescent suicide attempters. *Journal Of Clinical Child And Adolescent Psychology, 44*(1), 194–203. doi:10.1080/15374416.2014.940624

Asarnow, J. R., Hughes, J. L., Babeva, K. N., & Sugar, C. A. (2017). Cognitive-behavioral family treatment for suicide attempt prevention: A randomized controlled trial. *Journal of the American Academy of Child & Adolescent Psychiatry, 56*(6), 506–514. doi:10.1016/j.jaac.2017.03.015

Aseltine, R. J., & DeMartino, R. (2004). An outcome evaluation of the SOS suicide prevention program. *American Journal of Public Health, 94*(3), 446–451. doi:10.2105/ajph.94.3.446

Bauman, S., Toomey, R. B., & Walker, J. L. (2013). Associations among bullying, cyberbullying, and suicide in high school students. *Journal of Adolescence, 36*, 341–350. doi:10.1016/j.adolescence.2012.12.001

Brent, D., Greenhill, L., Compton, S., Emslie, G., Wells, K., Walkup, J., ... Turner, J. B. (2009). The treatment of adolescent suicide attempters (TASA) study: Predictors of suicidal events in an open treatment trial. *Journal of the American Academy of Child and Adolescent Psychiatry, 48*(10), 987–996. doi:10.1097/CHI.0b013e3181b5dbe4

Bridge, J., Horowitz, L., Fontanella, C., Sheftall, A. H., Greenhouse, J., Kelleher, K. J., ... Campo. J.V. (2018). Age-related racial disparity in suicide rates among US youths from 2001 through 2015. *JAMA Pediatrics*. doi: 10.1001/jamapediatrics.2018.0399.

Bridge, J. A., Asti, L., Horowitz, L. M., Greenhouse, J. B., Fontanella, C. A., Sheftall, A. H., ..., & Campo, J. V. (2015). Suicide trends among elementary school-aged children in the United States from 1993 to 2012. *JAMA Pediatrics*, *169*(7), 673–677. doi:10.1001/jamapediatrics.2015.0465

Bronfenbrenner, U. (1977). Toward an experimental ecology of human development. *American Psychologist*, *32*(7), 513–531. doi:10.1037/0003-066X.32.7.513

Bryan, C., Stone, S. L., & Rudd, M. D. (2011). A practical, evidence-based approach for means-restriction counseling with suicidal patients. *Professional Psychology: Research and Practice*, *42*, 339–346. doi:10.1037/a0025051

Cardeli, E. (2015). *Characteristics and functions of suicide attempts versus non-suicidal self-injury in juvenile confinement* (Unpublished doctoral dissertation), The Catholic University of America, Washington, DC.

Cash, S. J., & Bridge, J. A. (2009). Epidemiology of youth suicide and suicidal behavior. *Current Opinion in Pediatrics*, *21*(5), 613. doi:10.1097/MOP.0b013e32833063e1

Centers for Disease Control and Prevention. (2016). *Web-based injury statistics query and reporting system* [Data file]. Retrieved from https://www.cdc.gov/injury/wisqars/fatal.html.

Cha, C. B., Franz, P. J. M., Guzmán, E., Glenn, C. R., Kleiman, E. M., & Nock, M. K. (2018). Annual research review: Suicide among youth – Epidemiology, (potential) etiology, and treatment. *Journal Of Child Psychology And Psychiatry*, *59*(4), 460–482. doi:10.1111/jcpp.12831

Comtois, K. A., Jobes, D. A., O'Connor, S., Atkins, D. C., Janis, K., Chessen, C., ... Yuodelis Flores, C. (2011). Collaborative assessment and management of suicidality (CAMS): Feasibility trial for next-day appointment services. *Depression and Anxiety*, *28*, 963–972. doi:10.1002/da.20895

Connell, A. M., McKillop, H. N., & Dishion, T. J. (2016). Long-term effects of the family check-up in early adolescence on risk of suicide in early adulthood. *Suicide and Life-Threatening Behavior*, *46*(Suppl 1), S15–S22. doi:10.1111/sltb.2016.46.issue-S1

Conrad, A. K., Jacoby, A. M., Jobes, D. A., Lineberry, T., Jobes, D., Shea, C., ... Arnold-Ewing, T. (2009). A psychometric investigation of the suicide status form with suicidal inpatients. *Suicide and Life-Threatening Behavior*, *39*, 307–320. doi:10.1521/suli.2009.39.3.307

Curtin, S. C., Warner, M., & Hedegaard, H. (2016). Increase in suicide in the United States, 1999-2014. *NCHS Data Brief*, *241*, 1–8.

Czyz, E. K., Berona, M. S., & King, C. A. (2016). Rehospitalization of suicidal adolescents in relation to course of suicidal ideation and future suicide attempts. *Psychiatric Services*, *67*, 332–338. doi:10.1176/appi.ps.201400252

Diamond, G. S., Reis, B. F., Diamond, G. M., Siqueland, L., & Isaacs, L. (2002). Attachment-based family therapy for depressed adolescents: A treatment development study. *Journal of the American Academy of Child & Adolescent Psychiatry*, *41*, 1190–1196. doi:10.1097/00004583-200210000-00008

Diamond, G. S., Wintersteen, M. B., Brown, G. K., Diamond, G. M., Gallop, R., Shelef, K., & Levy, S. (2010). Attachment-based family therapy for adolescents with suicidal ideation: A randomized controlled trial. *Journal of the American Academy of Child & Adolescent Psychiatry*, *49*, 122–131.

Donaldson, D., Spirito, A., & Esposito-Smythers, C. (2005). Treatment for adolescents following a suicide attempt: Results of a pilot trial. *Journal of the American Academy of Child & Adolescent Psychiatry*, *44*, 113–120. doi:10.1097/00004583-200502000-00003

Esposito-Smythers, C., Spirito, A., Kahler, C. W., Hunt, J., & Monti, P. (2011). Treatment of co-occurring substance abuse and suicidality among adolescents: A randomized trial. *Journal of Consulting and Clinical Psychology*, *79*, 728. doi:10.1037/a0026074

Gilman, R., & Chard, K. (2015). Cognitive-behavioral and behavioral approaches. In H. T. Prout & A. L. Fedewa (Eds.), *Counseling and psychotherapy with children and adolescents: Theory and practice for school and clinical settings* (pp. 115-153). Hoboken, NJ: Wiley& Sons.

Glenn, C. R., Franklin, J. C., & Nock, M. K. (2015). Evidence-based psychosocial treatments for self-injurious thoughts and behaviors in youth. *Journal of Clinical Child and Adolescent Psychology, 44*, 1–29. doi:10.1080/15374416.2014.945211

Glenn, C. R., Lanzillo, E. C., Esposito, E. C., Santee, A. C., Nock, M. K., & Auerback, R. P. (2017). Examining the course of suicidal and non-suicidal self-injurious thoughts and behaviors In outpatient and inpatient adolescents. *Journal of Abnormal Child Psychology, 45*(971), 983. doi:10.1007/s10802-016-0214-0

Gosnell, S. N., Velasquez, K. M., Molfese, D., Molfese, P. J., Madan, A., Fowler, J. C., ... Salas, R. (2016). Prefrontal cortex, temporal cortex, and hippocampus volume are affected in suicidal psychiatric patients. *Psychiatry Research: Neuroimaging, 256*, 50–56. doi:10.1016/j.pscychresns.2016.09.005

Gould, M. S., & Lake, A. M. (2013). *The contagion of suicidal behavior* [Forum on Global Violence Prevention]. Retrieved from https://www.ncbi.nlm.nih.gov/books/NBK207262/.

Gould, M. S., Wallenstein, S., & Davidson, L. (1989). Suicide clusters: A critical review. *Suicide and Life-Threatening Behavior, 19*(1), 17–29.

Harrington, R., Kerfoot, M., Dyer, E., McNiven, F., Gill, J., Harrington, V., ... Byford, S. (1998). Randomized trial of a home-based family intervention for children who have deliberately poisoned themselves. *Journal of the American Academy of Child and Adolescent Psychiatry, 37*, 512–518. doi:10.1016/S0890-8567(14)60001-0

Hatzenbuehler, M. L. (2011). The social environment and suicide attempts in lesbian, gay, and bisexual youth. *Pediatrics, 127*, 896–903. doi:10.1542/peds.2010-3020

Hinduja, S., & Patchin, J. W. (2010). Bullying, cyberbullying, and suicide. *Archives of Suicide Research, 14*, 206–221. doi:10.1080/13811118.2010.494133

Huey, Jr, S. J., Henggeler, S. W., Rowland, M. D., Halliday-Boykins, C. A., Cunningham, P. B., & Pickrel, S. G. (2005). Predictors of treatment response for suicidal youth referred foremergency psychiatric hospitalization. *Journal of Clinical Childand Adolescent Psychology, 34*(3), 582–589. doi: 10.1207/s15374424jccp3403_13

Huh, D., Jobes, D. A., Comtois, K. A., Kerbrat, A. H., Chalker, S. A., Gutierrez, P. M., & Jennings, K. W. (2018). The Collaborative Assessment and Management of Suicidality (CAMS) versus Enhanced Care as Usual (E-CAU) with suicidal soldiers: Moderator analyses from a randomized controlled trial. *Military Psychology, 30*, 495–506. doi:10.1080/08995605.2018.1503001

Jobes, D. A. (2000). Collaborating to prevent suicide. *Suicide and Life-Threatening Behavior, 30*, 8–17.

Jobes, D. A. (2006). *Managing suicidal risk: A collaborative approach.* New York, NY: Guilford Press.

Jobes, D. A. (2012). The collaborative assessment and management of suicidality (CAMS): An evolving evidence-based clinical approach to suicidal risk. *Suicide and Life-Threatening Behavior, 42*, 640–653. doi:10.1111/j.1943-278X.2012.00119.x

Jobes, D. A. (2016). *Managing suicidal risk: A collaborative approach.* New York, NY: Guilford Publications.

Jobes, D. A., Au, J. S., & Siegelman, A. (2015). Psychological approaches to suicide treatment and prevention. *Current Treatment Options in Psychiatry, 2*(4), 363–370. doi:10.1007/s40501-015-0064-3

Jobes, D. A., Berman, A. L., & Josselson, A. R. (1987). Improving the validity and reliability of medicolegal certifications of suicide. *Suicide and Life-Threatening Behavior, 17*, 310–323.

Jobes, D. A., Comtois, K. A., Gutierrez, P. M., Brenner, L. A., Huh, D., Chalker, S. A., … Crow, B. (2017). A randomized controlled trial of the collaborative assessment and management of suicidality versus enhanced care as usual with suicidal soldiers. *Psychiatry: Interpersonal and Biological Processes*, *80*, 339–356. doi:10.1080/ 00332747.2017.1354607

Jobes, D. A., Gregorian, M. J., & Colborn, V. A. (2018). A stepped care approach to clinical suicide prevention. *Psychological Services*, *15*, 243–250. doi:10.1037/ser0000229

Jobes, D. A., Jacoby, A. M., Cimbolic, P., & Hustead, L. A. T. (1997). The assessment and treatment of suicidal clients in a university counseling center. *Journal of Counseling Psychology*, *44*, 368–377. doi:10.1037/0022-0167.44.4.368

Joiner, T. E., Sachs-Ericsson, N. J., Wingate, L. R., Brown, J. S., Anestis, M. D., & Selby, E. A. (2007). Childhood physical and sexual abuse and lifetime number of suicide attempts: A persistent and theoretically important relationship. *Behaviour Research and Therapy*, *45* (3), 539–547. doi:10.1016/j.brat.2006.04.007

Jokinen, J., Forslund, K., Ahnemark, E., Gustavsson, J. P., Nordström, P., & Åsberg, M. (2010). Karolinska interpersonal violence scale predicts suicide in suicide attempters. *The Journal of Clinical Psychiatry*. doi:10.4088/JCP.09m05944blu

Jollant, F., Bellivier, F., Leboyer, M., Astruc, B., Torres, S., Verdier, R., … Courtet, P. (2005). Impaired decision making in suicide attempters. *American Journal of Psychiatry*, *162*(2), 304–310. doi:10.1176/appi.ajp.162.2.304

Joshi, S. V., Hartley, S. N., Kessler, M., & Barstead, M. (2015). School-based suicide prevention: Content, process, and the role of trusted adults and peers. *Child and Adolescent Psychiatric Clinics*, *24*(2), 353–370. doi:10.1016/j.chc.2014.12.003

Katz, C., Bolton, S-L., Katz, L. Y., Isaak, C., Tilston-Jones, T., Sareen, J., & Swampy Cree Suicide Prevention Team. (2013). A systematic review of school-based suicide prevention programs. *Depression and Anxiety*, *30*, 1030–1045.

Klomek, A. B., Sourander, A., Niemela, S., Kumpulainen, K., Piha, J., Tamminen, T., … Gould, M. S. (2009). Childhood bullying behaviors as a risk for suicide attempts and completed suicides: A population-based birth cohort study. *Journal of the American Academy of Child and Adolescent Psychiatry*, *48*, 254–261. doi:10.1097/CHI.0b013e318196b91f

Lanzillo, E. C., Horowitz, L. M., & Pao, M. (2018). Suicide in Children. In T. Falcone & J. Timmon Mitchell (Eds.). *Suicide prevention: A practical guide for the practitioner* (pp. 73–107). doi:10.1007/978-3-319-74391-2

Large, M., Ryan, C., Walsh, G., Stein-Parbury, J., & Patfield, M. (2014). Nosocomial suicide. *Australian Psychiatry*, *22*, 118–121. doi:10.1177/1039856213511277

Linehan, M. (1993). *Cognitive behavioral treatment of borderline personality disorder*. New York, NY: Guilford.

Liu, R. T., & Miller, I. (2014). Life events and suicidal ideation and behavior: A systematic review. *Clinical Psychology Review*, *34*(3), 181–192. doi:10.1016/j.cpr.2014.01.006

McCauley, E., Berk, M. S., Asarnow, J. R., Adrian, M., Cohen, J., Korslund, K., … Linehan, M. M. (2018). Efficacy of Dialectical Behavior Therapy for adolescents at high risk for suicide: A randomized clinical trial. *JAMA Psychiatry (Chicago, Ill.)*, *75*(8), 777–785. doi:10.1001/jamapsychiatry.2018.1109

Mehlum, L., Ramberg, M., Tørmoen, A. J., Haga, E., Diep, L. M., Stanley, B. H., … Grøholt, B. (2016). Dialectical behavior therapy compared with enhanced usual care for adolescents with repeated suicidal and self-harming behavior: Outcomes over a one-year follow-up. *Journal of the American Academy of Child and Adolescent Psychiatry*, *55*, 295–300. doi:10.1016/j.jaac.2016.01.005

Mehlum, L., Tørmoen, A. J., Ramberg, M., Haga, E., Diep, L. M., Laberg, S., … Grøholt, B. (2014). Dialectical behavior therapy for adolescents with repeated suicidal and self-harming behavior: A randomized trial. *Journal of the American Academy of Child and Adolescent Psychiatry, 53*, 1082–1091. doi:10.1016/j.jaac.2014.07.003

Michael, K. D., & Jameson, J. P. (2017). *Handbook of rural school mental health.* New York, NY: Springer.

Michael, K. D., Jameson, J. P., Filbin, B., Rosston, K., & Butts, E. (2017, April). Creating multiple paths for effective risk management: Making MTSS (Multi-tiered systems of Support) work for suicide prevention in schools. Paper presented at the Annual Convention of the American Association of Suicidology. Phoenix, Arizona.

Miller, A. L., Rathus, J. H., Linehan, M. M., Wetzler, S., & Leigh, E. (1997). Dialectical behavior therapy adapted for suicidal adolescents. *Journal of Psychiatric Practice, 3*(2), 78. doi:10.1097/00131746-199703000-00002

National Action Alliance for Suicide Prevention: Transforming Health Systems Initiative Work Group. (2018). *Recommended standard care for people with suicide risk: Making healthcare suicide safe.* Washington, DC: Education Development Center.

Nock, M. K., & Banaji, M. R. (2007). Prediction of suicide ideation and attempts among adolescents using a brief performance-based test. *Journal of Consulting and Clinical Psychology, 75*(5), 707. doi:10.1037/0022-006X.75.5.707

Nock, M. K., Borges, G., Bromet, E. J., Cha, C. B., Kessler, R. C., & Lee, S. (2008). Suicide and suicidal behavior. *Epidemiologic Reviews, 30*(1), 133–154. doi: 10.1093/epirev/mxn002

Nock, M. K., Green, J. G., Hwang, I., McLaughlin, K. A., Sampson, N. A., Zaslavsky, A. M., & Kessler, R. C. (2013). Prevalence, correlates, and treatment of lifetime suicidal behavior among adolescents: Results from the National Comorbidity Survey Replication adolescent supplement lifetime suicidal behavior among adolescents. *JAMA Psychiatry (Chicago, Ill.), 70*, 300–310. doi:10.1001/2013.jamapsychiatry.55

Nock, M. K., & Kazdin, A. E. (2002). Examination of affective, cognitive, and behavioral factors and suicide-related outcomes in children and young adolescents. *Journal of Clinical Child and Adolescent Psychology, 31*, 48–58. doi:10.1207/S15374424JCCP3101_07

O'Connor, S. S., Brausch, A., Ridge-Anderson, A., & Jobes, D. A. (2014). Applying the collaborative assessment and management of suicidality (CAMS) to suicidal adolescents. *International Journal of Behavioral Consultation and Therapy, 9*, 53–58. doi:10.1037/h0101641

Ordaz, S. J., Goyer, M. S., Ho, T. C., Singh, M. K., & Gotlib, I. H. (2018). Network basis of suicidal ideation in depressed adolescents. *Journal of Affective Disorders, 226*, 92–99. doi:10.1016/j.jad.2017.09.021

Ougrin, D., Tranah, T., Stahl, D., Moran, P., & Asarnow, J. R. (2015). Therapeutic interventions for suicide attempts and self-harm in adolescents: Systematic review and meta-analysis. *Journal Of The American Academy Of Child & Adolescent Psychiatry, 54* (2), 97–107. doi:10.1016/j.jaac.2014.10.009

Pao, M., Jobes, D., Falcone, T., Timmons-Mitchell, J., Horowitz, L., & Austerman, J. (2017, October). *Clinical perspectives on suicide prevention.* Panel presented at the 64th Annual Meeting of the American Academy of Child and Adolescent Psychiatry, Washington, DC.

Perepletchikova, F., Axelrod, S. R., Kaufman, J., Rounsaville, B. J., Douglas-Palumberi, H., & Miller, A. L. (2011). Adapting dialectical behaviour therapy for children: Towards a new research agenda for pediatric suicidal and non-suicidal self-injurious behaviours. *Child and Adolescent Mental Health, 16*, 116–121. doi:10.1111/j.1475-3588.2010.00583.x

Pfeffer, C. (1986). *The suicidal child.* New York, NY: Guilford Press.

Plemmons, G., Hall, M., Doupnik, S., Gay, J., Brown, C., Browning, W., ... & Rehm, K. (2018). Hospitalization for suicide ideation or attempt: 2008–2015. *Pediatrics, 141*(6). doi:10.1542/peds.2017-2426

Plunkett, A., O'Toole, B., Swanston, H., Oates, R. K., Shrimpton, S., & Parkinson, P. (2001). Suicide risk following child sexual abuse. *Ambulatory Pediatrics, 1*(5), 262–266.

Poston, J. M., & Hanson, W. E. (2010). Meta-analysis of psychological assessment as a therapeutic intervention. *Psychological Assessment, 22,* 203–210. doi:10.1037/a0018679

Powers, J. T., Brausch, A. M., McClay, M. M., Gregory, J. A., Miller, K. N., O'Connor, S. S., & Jobes, D. A. (2018, April). Relationships between the Suicide Index Score, implicit suicide ideation, and reasons for living in a clinical sample of adolescents. Poster presented at the annual conference of the American Association of Suicidology, Washington, DC.

Rajalin, M., Hirvikoski, T., & Jokinen, J. (2013). Family history of suicide and exposure to interpersonal violence in childhood predict suicide in male suicide attempters. *Journal of Affective Disorders, 148*(1), 92–97. doi:10.1016/j.jad.2012.11.055

Rathus, J. H., & Miller, A. L. (2002). Dialectical behavior therapy adapted for suicidal adolescents. *Suicide and Life-Threatening Behavior, 32,* 146–157. doi:10.1521/suli.32.2.146.24399

Ridge-Anderson, A., Jobes, D. A., & Lento, R. M. (2017, June). *Treating suicidality in older adolescents.* Poster presented at the Journal of Clinical Child and Adolescent Psychology, Future Directions Forum, College Park, Maryland.

Ridge-Anderson, A., Keyes, G. M., & Jobes, D. A. (2016). Understanding and treating suicidal risk in young children. *Practice Innovations, 1,* 3–19. doi:10.1037/pri0000018

Robertson, L., Skegg, K., Poore, M., Williams, S., & Taylor, B. (2012). An adolescent suicide cluster and the possible role of electronic communication technology. *Crisis, 33*(4), 239–245. doi:10.1027/0227-5910/a000140

Robinson, J., Cox, G., Malone, A., Williamson, M., Baldwin, G., Fletcher, K., & O'Brien, M. (2013). A systematic review of school-based interventions aimed at preventing, treating, and responding to suicide-related behavior in young people. *Crisis: the Journal of Crisis Intervention and Suicide Prevention, 34,* 164. doi:10.1027/0227-5910/a000168

Rodway, C., Tham, S. G., Ibrahim, S., Turnbull, P., Windfuhr, K., Shaw, J., … Appleby, L. (2016). Suicide in children and young people in England: A consecutive case series. *The Lancet Psychiatry, 3*(8), 751–759. doi:10.1016/S2215-0366(16)30094-3

Romanowicz, M., O'Connor, S. S., Schak, K. M., Swintak, C. C., & Lineberry, T. W. (2013). Use of the Suicide Status Form-II to investigate correlates of suicide risk factors in psychiatrically hospitalized children and adolescents. *Journal of Affective Disorders, 151* (2), 467–473. doi:10.1016/j.jad.2013.06.026

Rosin, H. (2015). The Silicon Valley Suicides: Why are so many kids with bright prospects killing themselves in Palo Alto? *The Atlantic.* Retrieved from https://www.theatlantic.com/magazine/archive/2015/12/the-silicon-valleysuicides/413140/.

Salzinger, S., Rosario, M., Feldman, R. S., & Ng-Mak, D. S. (2007). Adolescent suicidal behavior: Associations with preadolescent physical abuse and selected risk and protective factors. *Journal of the American Academy of Child & Adolescent Psychiatry, 46*(7), 859 866. doi:10.1097/chi.0b013e318054e702

Sandler, I., Tein, J.-Y., Wolchik, S., & Ayers, T. S. (2016). The effects of the family bereavement program to reduce suicide ideation and/or attempts of parentally bereaved children six and fifteen years later. *Suicide and Life-Threatening Behavior, 46*(Suppl 1), S32–S38. doi:10.1111/sltb.2016.46.issue-S1

Scelfo, J. (2015, August 5). Suicide on campus and the pressure of perfection. *The New York Times.* Retrieved from https://www.nytimes.com/2015/08/02/education/edlife/stresssocial-media-and-suicide-on-campus.html

Schembari, B. C., Jobes, D. A., & Horgan, R. (2016). Successful treatment of suicidal risk: What helped and what was internalized? *Crisis: the Journal of Crisis Intervention and Suicide Prevention.* doi:10.1027/0227-5910/a000370

Schilling, E. A., Lawless, M., Buchanan, L., & Aseltine, R. J. (2014). 'Signs of Suicide' shows promise as a middle school suicide prevention program. *Suicide And Life-Threatening Behavior, 44*(6), 653–667. doi:10.1111/sltb.12097

Sheftall, A. H., Asti, L., Horowitz, L. M., Felts, A., Fontanella, C. A., Campo, J. V., & Bridge, J. A. (2016). Suicide in elementary school-aged children and adolescents. *Pediatrics, 138*, pii: e20160436. doi:10.1542/peds.2016-0436

Spirito, A., Esposito-Smythers, C., & Wolff, J. (2018). Developing and testing interventions for suicidal and non-suicidal self-injury among adolescents. In J. R. Weisz & A. E. Kazdin (Eds.), *Evidence-based psychotherapies for children and adolescents.* (3rd ed., pp. 235–252). New York, NY: Guilford Press.

Stanley, I. H., Horowitz, L. M., Bridge, J. A., Wharff, E. A., & Teach, S. J. (2016). Bullying and suicide risk among pediatric emergency department patients. *Pediatric Emergency Care, 32* (6), 347. doi:10.1097/PEC.0000000000000537

Tang, T. C., Jou, S. H., Ko, C. H., Huang, S. Y., & Yen, C. F. (2009). Randomized study of school-based intensive interpersonal psychotherapy for depressed adolescents with suicidal risk and parasuicide behaviors. *Psychiatry and Clinical Neurosciences, 63*, 463–470. doi:10.1111/j.1440-1819.2009.01991.x

Van Geel, M., Vedder, P., & Tanilon, J. (2014). Relationship between peer victimization, cyberbullying, and suicide in children and adolescents: A meta-analysis. *JAMA Pediatrics, 168*, 435–442. doi:10.1001/jamapediatrics.2013.4143

Vergara, G. A., Stewart, J. G., Cosby, E. A., Lincoln, S. H., & Auerbach, R. P. (2019). Non-suicidal self-injury and suicide in depressed adolescents: Impact of peer victimization and bullying. *Journal of Affective Disorders, 245*, 744–749. doi:10.1016/j.jad.2018.11.084

Wagner, B. M. (1997). Family risk factors for child and adolescent suicidal behavior. *Psychological Bulletin, 121*, 246–298.

Wyman, P. A., Brown, C. H., LoMurray, M., Schmeelk-Cone, K., Petrova, M., Yu, Q., & Wang, W. (2010). An outcome evaluation of the Sources of Strength suicide prevention program delivered by adolescent peer leaders in high schools. *American Journal of Public Health, 100*, 1653–1661. doi:10.2105/AJPH.2009.190025

Zhang, S., Chen, J. M., Kuang, L., Cao, J., Zhang, H., Ai, M., … Fang, W. D. (2016). Association between abnormal default mode network activity and suicidality in depressed adolescents. *BMC Psychiatry, 16*, 227. doi:10.1186/s12888-016-1047-7

Index

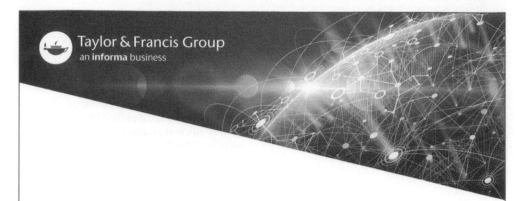
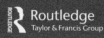
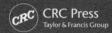